# DOPPLER APPLICATIONS IN LEO SATELLITE COMMUNICATION SYSTEMS

***CD-Rom Included***

# THE KLUWER INTERNATIONAL SERIES IN ENGINEERING AND COMPUTER SCIENCE

# DOPPLER APPLICATIONS IN LEO SATELLITE COMMUNICATION SYSTEMS

***CD-Rom Included***

**Irfan Ali**
*Motorola, Global Telecom Solutions Sector*

**Pierino G. Bonanni**
*GE Corporate Research & Development*

**Naofal Al-Dhahir**
*AT&T Shannon Laboratory*

**John E. Hershey**
*GE Corporate Research & Development*

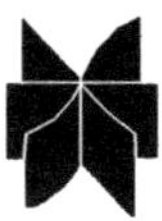

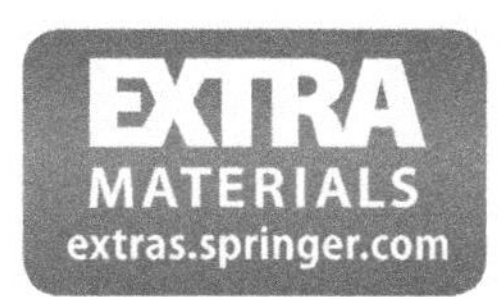


SPRINGER SCIENCE+BUSINESS MEDIA, LLC

DOI 10.1007/978-0-306-47546-7

**Additional material to this book can be downloaded from http://extras.springer.com**

---

**Library of Congress Cataloging-in-Publication Data**

A C.I.P. Catalogue record for this book is available
from the Library of Congress.

---


Originally published by Kluwer Academic Publishers in 2002

MyCopy version of the original edition 2002



*Printed on acid-free paper.*
www.springer.com/mycopy

*To my parents, Zarrin and Rustam Ali.*
Irfan Ali

*To my wife, Julie, and to our greatest joy, Matthew.*
Pierino Bonanni

*To my wife, Alia, for her unconditional love and support.*
Naofal Al-Dhahir

*To two great friends and teachers, Amer Hassan and Rao Yarlagadda.*
John Hershey

# Contents

# Preface

This book is about making a virtue out of a necessity. More specifically, it is about harnessing the very significant Doppler shifts encountered in communications involving Earth stations and low Earth orbit (LEO) satellites as an aid to those communications. We have come to believe that very real benefits may be easily derived from Doppler shift signal processing and analysis for communications flow control and power control. What makes Doppler especially attractive from an implementation point of view is the generally implied necessity to measure it for other reasons, most notably the need to pre- or post-compensate for the Doppler shift on the communications processing chain. Thus, most communications terminals will have a voltage somewhere that can be accessed and discretized and serve as the Doppler input to our algorithms and methods.

The book has been set into seven chapters. The first chapter is a recounting of the characteristics of a LEO satellite and its orbit, and a brief sampling of the already rich history of the art, as reflected by various LEO satellites and their missions. Chapter two addresses the LEO orbital geometry and reviews the Doppler effect in LEO communications. Chapter three is concerned with the important task of estimating the Doppler at a ground terminal. Appropriate signal processing algorithms are reviewed. Chapter four is concerned with predicting LEO satellite visibility. Chapters five and six are, respectively, devoted to the use of the significant LEO Doppler as an aid in traffic flow control and as an aid for effecting communications power control.

Chapter 7 describes MATLAB® based analysis and demonstration software that we have chosen to provide with the book. The software is, first, a collection of functions useful for calculating satellite orbits, terrestrial contours and regions, and coordinate transformations based on Earth rotation. They are functions that have proven fundamental to the analysis of the DBMA protocol described in the book. Second, the software includes a set of user-friendly graphical animation routines that aid in visualization of a LEO orbit, its coverage regions, and the DBMA concept.

The authors would like to acknowledge the GE Corporate Research and Development Center for giving us the opportunity to investigate LEO satellites. We would also like to thank Mr. John Paffett of the Surrey Space Centre for permission to use some materials in Chapter 1. Finally, we would like to thank our wives – Özden, Julie, Alia and Anna – for their love and patience.

Irfan Ali

Pierino G. Bonanni

Naofal Al-Dhahir

John E. Hershey

# Chapter 1

# Little LEO Satellites

In this chapter we qualitatively salute the value of a low Earth orbit (LEO) satellite's orbit. We review the history of LEO satellite deployment with brief and edited summarization. We then proceed to review LEO satellite orbits, coordinate reference frames, and other conventions and aids essential for determining a satellite's orbit from the perspective of an observer on the Earth's surface. As will be evident, the single most striking feature of LEO communications is the significant Doppler shift encountered by virtue of the rapid dynamics of the low Earth orbit. It is the goal of this book to show how to make good use of this feature that at first blush appears to a communications engineer as a pesky problem complicating synchronization and requiring added complexity in various tracking loops.

## 1. THE LEO AND ITS VALUE

Partition in LEO satellites appears first in satellite complexity or size, giving rise to the terms "Big LEO" and "Little LEO." The Little LEOs are those satellites that handle relatively short data messages that are not time critical. Little LEO satellites are not cross-linked through space, and may function in either a "bent pipe" transponder mode or as message store-and-forward data transportation vehicles. Little LEOs are almost always in circular orbits and they may or may not use stationkeeping. Little LEO orbits have been proposed with very different inclinations, the angle formed between the orbit plane and the equatorial plane. In some cases these inclinations are specifically chosen to optimize customer service requirements, in other cases the inclination is essentially a result of a major satellite launch on which the Little LEO piggybacked.

Little LEO satellites are physically small, generally single mission satellites operating without sophisticated measures such as the previously stated direct satellite-to-satellite cross-linking, and are relatively inexpensive to build and to launch. For communications services, which is the motivation behind this work, they are generally employed as a set of identical satellites regularly positioned about a series of orbital planes in order that line-of-sight services to specific areas on the Earth are in accordance with some system specification such as a maximum time that a ground station must wait until a satellite is in view above a minimum elevation angle. The Low Earth Orbit is not a hard and fast specification. Sturza [1] offers a reasonable characterization however: "Low Earth Orbits are generally considered to be those with altitudes between 500 km and 2,000 km. Lower altitudes [result] in quick re-entry and higher altitudes are subject to severe radiation from the Van Allen Belts." Table 1 is a sampling of Little LEO projects for communications. It was developed from data placed on the Web by SSTL [2].

*Table 1.* A sampling of actual and proposed Little LEO satellite projects for communications reasearch and services.

| Satellite Name | Date of Launch | Orbit (km) | Inclina tion (deg) | Communication Mission |
|---|---|---|---|---|
| OSCAR-6 | 10/15/72 | 1453x1447 | 101.4 | Rad. Am. Sat. Three transponders one of which "Codestore" allowed Morse & teletype to be stored & retransmitted |
| RS-1 & RS-2 | 10/26/78 | 1689x1709 | 82.55 | Russian Rad. Am. Sat. Transponders and "Codestore"-like unit |
| UoSAT-2 (OSCAR-11) | 3/1/84 | 679x697 | 98.25 | First operational digital S&F comm. payload |
| GLOMR | 10/26/85 | 326 | 57 | S&F comm. |
| UoSAT-3 (OSCAR-14, VITASAT, HealthSat-1) | 1/22/90 | 780 | 98 | S&F @ 9600 bps. |
| OSCAR-16 (PacSAT) | 1/22/90 | 780 | 98 | Am. Digital S&F packet data @ 1200 bps. |
| OSCAR-18 (WeberSat) | 1/22/90 | 780 | 98 | Digital S&F packet comm. |
| OSCAR-19 (LuSAT) | 1/22/90 | 780 | 98 | Digital S&F packet comm. |
| Fuji-2 | 2/7/90 | - | - | Analog comm. transponders |
| TECEL/SECS | 4/5/90 | 489x668 | 94.1 | Comm. Experiments. S&F data relay. |
| MACSAT-1 | 5/9/90 | 608x766 | 89.9 | S&F data comm. Multiple Access Comm. Sats. |

| Satellite Name | Date of Launch | Orbit (km) | Inclina tion (deg) | Communication Mission |
|---|---|---|---|---|
| BADR-A | 7/16/90 | - | - | S&F transponder in 144-146 MHz & 435-436 MHz bands. |
| MicroSats | 7/16/91 | 359x457 (833x833 intended) | 82 | Bent pipe relay for many comm. Traffics. Limited S&F. |
| UoSAT-5 (OSCAR-22) | 7/17/91 | - | - | Digital S&F comm. Am. Sat. service research testbed for LEO comm. protocols |
| TUBSAT-1 | 7/17/91 | - | - | Test 1.5/1.6 GHz data relay system. |
| KitSat-1 (OSCAR-23) | 8/10/92 | 1328x1316 | 66 | Rad. Am. Digital S&F transponder. |
| S80/T | 8/10/92 | 1338x1315 | 66.1 | Characterize radio environment from 148-149.9 MHz |
| OXP-1 | 2/9/93 | 722x787 | 24.97 | Determine global VHF frequency utilization |
| RADCAL | 6/25/93 | 765x884 | 89.5 | UHF S&F payload |
| TemiSAT | 8/30/93 | 980x945 | 82.5 | Uplink & Downlink weather data. S&F transponder |
| PoSAT-1 | 9/26/93 | 822x800 | 98.6 | Experimental communications DSP. Email. |
| ItamSat | 9/26/93 | 823x799 | 98.6 | Am. Digital S&F Comm. |
| Health-Sat-2 | 9/26/93 | 821x797 | 98.6 | Relay of emergency medical information |
| EyeSat | 9/26/93 | 823x794 | 98.5 | Digital S&F transponder |
| RS-15A (RADIO-ROSTO) | 12/16/94 | 2165x1885 | 64.6 | Linear comm. transponders |
| JAS-2 | 8/17/96 | 797x1317 | 98.6 | Rad. Am. Sat. Linear transponder for SSB & CW |

A LEO satellite may have a distinct advantage over a geosynchronous orbit (GEO) satellite by virtue of the "elevation search" capability. As depicted in *Figure 1*, it is conceivable that a communications asset on the Earth will be shadowed and unable to communicate to a geostationary satellite. In the case shown, a building is obstructing the path from the transmitter to the GEO. As both the GEO and the transmitter are fixed, the path will remain blocked. Also shown is a LEO that moves with respect to the blocking building and the fixed transmitter. At first, the LEO path is similarly blocked. Later, however, the LEO moves into positions where the path is no longer blocked. Thus, a LEO, with its dynamic geometry, is often capable of allowing a link to be established which would be impossible for a fixed transmitter/GEO scenario.

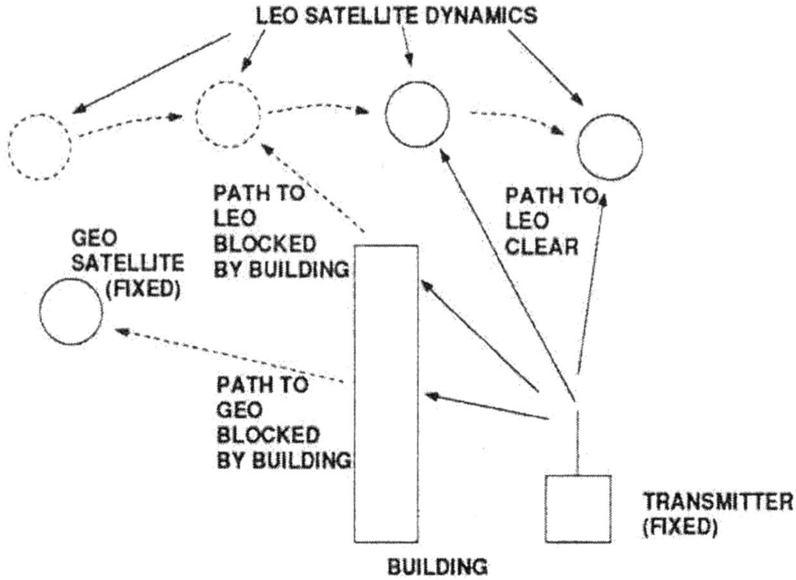


*Figure 1.* The value of the LEO satellite's dynamic geometry.

## 2. KEPLERIAN ELEMENTS

Keplerian parameters or elements define an orbit as an ellipse, orient the ellipse with respect to the Earth and then place a satellite at an instant of time on the ellipse. In the Keplerian model, satellites orbit the Earth in an ellipse of constant shape and orientation. In reality, perturbations due to Earth's shape, atmospheric drag, and gravitational pull of the sun and the moon cause the orbit to deviate from its ideal elliptical shape. We will not cover these perturbations in this chapter and in the book, as these perturbations cause higher order modifications to a satellite's orbit which are usually compensated by active stationkeeping. The reader should refer to books on satellite geometry that cover this topic in detail.

Though in this book we are only concerned with circular orbits that require fewer Keplerian elements to define, we will introduce all the Keplerian elements used to define an elliptical orbit. It is important for the reader to be aware of all these elements as these elements are commonly used in most textbooks on satellite communication.

A satellite orbit is an ellipse with one focus, $f_1$, at the Earth's center as sketched in *Figure 2* wherein:

$f_1$ and $f_2$ are the foci,

$r_E$ is the radius of the Earth, $r_E = 6378$ km,

$h_p$ is the height above the Earth of the satellite's closest approach to the Earth called *perigee*,

$h_a$ is the height above the Earth of the satellite's farthest distance from the Earth called *apogee*,

$a$ is the length of the orbit's semi-major axis,

$b$ is the length of the orbit's semi-minor axis.

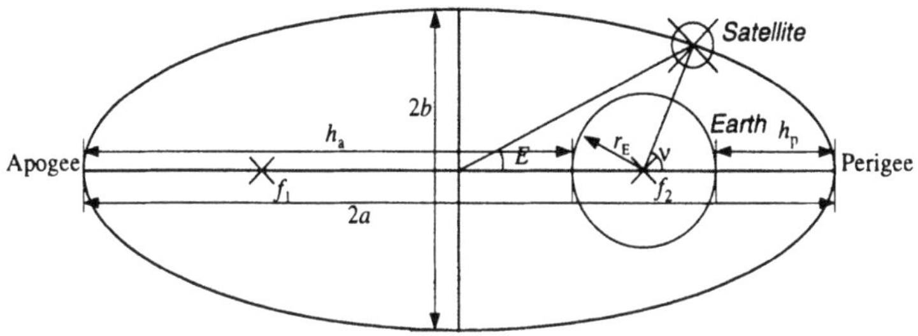


*Figure 2.* Satellite orbit ellipse.

The Keplerian elements used to describe an orbit and locate a satellite on the orbit are:

1. The *length of the semi-major axis, a*. The period of a satellite's orbit, $T$, the time, in seconds, required for a satellite to traverse one full path of its elliptical orbit, is

$$T = 2\pi\sqrt{\frac{a^3}{\mu}} \tag{1}$$

where $a$ is in km and $\mu = 398600.5\frac{km^3}{s^2}$. Another parameter associated with the semi-major axis is the mean motion, $n$

$$n = \frac{2\pi}{T} = \sqrt{\frac{\mu}{a^3}} \tag{2}$$

2. The *eccentricity*, $e$, which measures the ellipticity of the orbit is

$$e = \frac{h_a - h_p}{h_a + h_p + 2r_E} \tag{3}$$

If the satellite's orbit is circular, the apogee and perigee are the same and the eccentricity is zero.

3. The *inclination* of the orbital plane, $i$. This is the angle between the plane containing the satellite's orbit and the Earth's equatorial plane, as shown in *Figure 3*. There we see that the planes form intersection angles of $i$ degrees and 180-$i$ degrees. The ambiguity is resolved by picking the angle, $i$, which is formed when the satellite crosses from the Southern Hemisphere to the Northern Hemisphere. A right-hand convention is used. Curl the fingers of the right hand about the satellite orbit with the fingers pointing in the direction of the satellite's motion. Erect the thumb so that it is normal to the orbital plane. The thumb then forms an angle with the line joining the center of the Earth and the North Pole. An inclination of $90^0$ is termed a *polar orbit*.

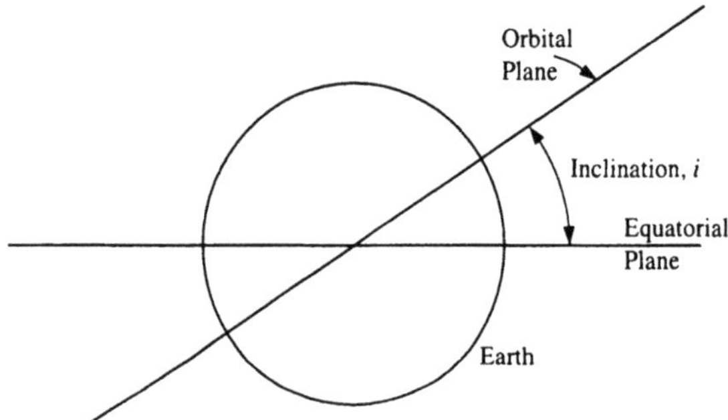


*Figure 3.* The inclination of a satellite orbit.

4. *Right ascension of the ascending node, Ω.* Two parameters are used to orient a satellite's orbital plane in space, the first of which is the inclination angle, $i$, and the second is the right ascension of ascending node. For a given inclination angle, there are infinite number of orbital plane orientations, with each orientation intersecting the equator at different points. The right ascension of ascending node fixes the intersection of the orbital plane with the equator and is shown in *Figure 4*. The orbital plane intersects the equator at two points. In one of the points the satellite is going from the south to the north hemisphere. This point is called the *ascending node*. The other point is called the *descending node*. The right ascension of the ascending node is the angle between the line joining the Earth's center to the ascending node and the line joining the Earth's center to the vernal equinox. Vernal equinox will be described in the next section. For the current moment, vernal equinox can be assumed to be a fixed point in space (which is not completely true,

but will suffice for the moment). If the right ascension of the ascending node is zero, the orbital plane crosses the equator at the line of vernal equinox.

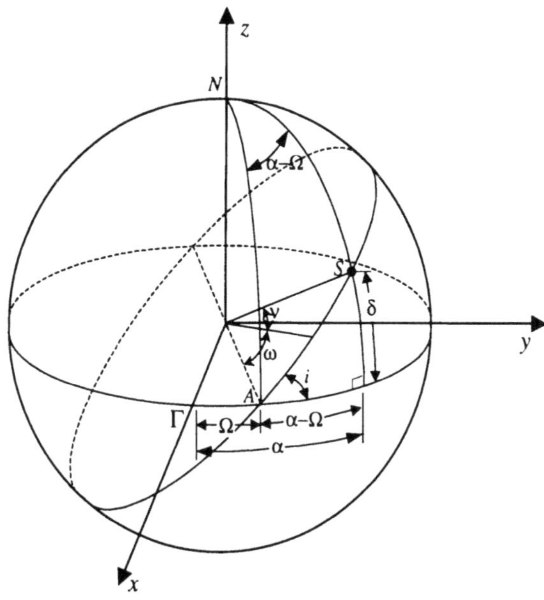


*Figure 4.* The orientation of a satellite's orbit [3].

5. *Argument of perigee, $\omega$.* Now that we have oriented the orbital plane in space, the next parameter, namely argument of perigee, is used to orient the satellite's orbit, especially an elliptical orbit, in the orbital plane. The argument of perigee is the angle from the ascending node to the perigee. The angle is measured counter-clockwise from the ascending node. For circular orbit satellites, this angle is undefined. However, accurately speaking, circular orbits are essentially elliptical orbits with a very small value of eccentricity. Hence, the argument of perigee is also defined for most circular orbits.
6. *Anomaly: Mean Anomaly (M), True Anomaly ($\nu$) and Eccentric Anomaly (E).* Anomaly is angle measurement used to define the location of a satellite in its orbit. *Mean anomaly* is an angle measurement that increases at a constant rate from 0 degrees to 360 degrees. It is defined to be zero when the satellite is at is perigee and it is 180 degrees when the satellite is at its apogee. For circular orbits, since the angular velocity of

the satellite is a constant, a line from the Earth's center at an angle equal to the mean anomaly from the line of perigee actually points at the location of the satellite in the orbit. For elliptical orbits, since the angular velocity of the satellite is not a constant, a line at mean anomaly angle from the perigee does not point at the satellite. True anomaly is the angle at the Earth's center between the satellite's current location and the line of perigee, as shown in *Figure 2* for elliptical orbit satellites. For circular orbits, true anomaly is equal to the mean anomaly. Another term, *eccentric anomaly*, is also used in orbital geometry, and it is shown in *Figure 2*.

The mean anomaly, $M$, at any time $t$ is defined as

$$M = \frac{2\pi}{T}(t - \tau) \tag{4}$$

where $T$ is the orbit period and $\tau$ is the time at perigee. The relation between the mean anomaly, true anomaly and eccentric anomaly is given below

$$\tan\frac{v}{2} = \sqrt{\frac{1+e}{1-e}}\tan\frac{E}{2} \tag{5}$$

$$M = E - e\sin E \tag{6}$$

$$v = M + \left(2e - \frac{e^3}{4}\right)\sin M + \frac{5}{4}e^2\sin 2M + \frac{13}{12}e^3\sin 3M + \cdots \tag{7}$$

$$\begin{aligned} E &= M + 2\sum_{k=1}^{\infty}\frac{1}{k}J_k(ke)\sin kM \\ &= M + e\sin M + \frac{e^2}{2}\sin 2M + \frac{e^3}{8}(3\sin 3M - \sin M) + \cdots \end{aligned} \tag{8}$$

The values of the three anomalies coincide when the satellite is at the perigee (value equals 0 degrees) and at the apogee (value equals 180 degrees).

Two parameters usually used to specify the location of a satellite in its orbit are the right ascension $\alpha$ and declination $\delta$, as shown in *Figure 4*. Applying the law of sines to the spherical triangle (i.e., triangle formed by arcs of great circles) *ASN*, we obtain,

$$\sin(\alpha - \Omega) = \frac{\cos i}{\cos \delta} \sin(\omega + \nu) \tag{9}$$

Also, from the law of cosines of sides applied to the spherical triangle *ABS*,

$$\cos(\omega + \nu) = \cos \delta \cos(\alpha - \Omega) \tag{10}$$

Eliminating cos $\delta$ from these two equations,

$$\tan(\alpha - \Omega) = \cos i \tan(\omega + \nu) \tag{11}$$

or,

$$\alpha = \arctan[\cos i \tan(\omega + \nu)] + \Omega \tag{12}$$

Also, by the law of sines,

$$\sin \delta = \sin i \sin(\omega + \nu) \tag{13}$$

or

$$\delta = \arcsin[\sin i \sin(\omega + \nu)] \tag{14}$$

The above six parameters define an orbit and a satellite's location in the orbit at a particular time.

A widely used format for distributing satellite orbit parameters is the so-called "NASA 2-line format" (actually three lines, with the first providing the name of the satellite). A Web site from which orbit parameters can be obtained in this form for most LEO satellites is [4]. An example of the NASA 2-line format for an Orbcomm satellite, downloaded from the Web site on August 20, 1999, is shown in *Figure 5*. There it is shown that each number is in a specific fixed column, and spaces are significant. The complete definition of all the information elements in the 2-line format is provided at the Web site [4].

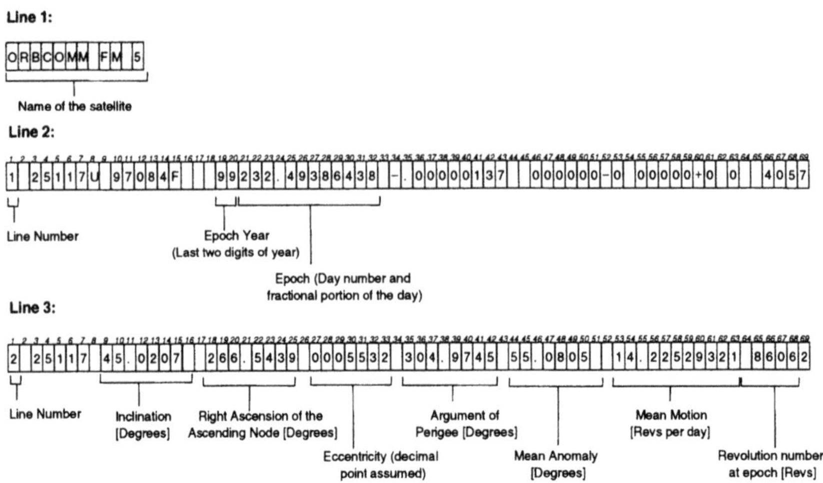


*Figure 5.* NASA 2-line format for orbital data.

The relevant orbital information for this Orbcomm satellite is given in *Table 2*.

*Table 2*. Orbcomm satellite data

| Parameter | Value |
|---|---|
| Year | 1991 |
| Calendar Day Number | 232 (August 20) |
| Time after 0.0 GMT | 0.49386438 (11:51:09.50) |
| Eccentricity, $e$ | 0.005532 |
| Inclination, $i$ | $45.0207^0$ |
| Argument of perigee, $\omega$ | $304.9745^0$ |
| Right ascension of ascending node, $\Omega$ | $266.5439^0$ |
| Mean anomaly, $M$ | $55.0805^0$ |
| Mean motion, $n$ | 14.22529321 rev/day |

## 3. REFERENCE FRAMES

Three reference frames are commonly used in orbital geometry, as each frame is well suited for representing a different set of geometric concepts. A reference frame fixed in space, the Earth-centered inertial (ECI) reference frame, is best used to specify the parameters of a satellite's orbit. A reference frame fixed to the Earth, the Earth-centered fixed (ECF) reference frame, is favored when it is desired to describe the location of a satellite in orbit in terms of geographic latitude and longitude. A reference frame centered on an observer on the Earth's surface, the topocentric reference frame, is best suited to determine quantities that determine the location of a satellite with respect to the user, such as elevation angle, slant range, and direction to the satellite. We will first describe the reference frames and then provide the transformations between reference frames.

## 3.1 Earth Centered Inertial (ECI) Reference Frame

This reference frame is centered at the Earth with the *x*-axis pointing towards a (quasi) fixed point in space – the *vernal equinox* – and the *z*-axis along the axis of rotation of the Earth.

The easiest way to define the vernal equinox, represented by the symbol ♈, is to consider the revolution of the Earth around the sun. From the perspective of the Earth, the sun can be assumed to rotate around the Earth. Consider for an instant the Earth to be stationary about its axis. Due to the 23.5-degree tilt of the Earth's equator with respect to the plane of the Earth's orbit around the sun, the trajectory of the sun's orbit with respect to Earth is "inclined" by 23.5 degrees from the equator. This inclination in more technical terms is the "obliquity of the ecliptic." On one particular day every year, the trajectory of the sun's orbit crosses the Earth's equator going from south to north. This day is called the "first day of Spring". The direction from the center of the Earth through the point of intersection of the sun's orbit with the equator is called the vernal equinox.

Had the sun been stationary in space, the vernal equinox would always be pointing to the same zodiac in space. In fact, about 3000 years ago, when Babylonians codified the zodiac, the vernal equinox was pointing to the Aries constellation; hence, the symbol ♈ denoting Aries and the reference to vernal equinox as the "first point of Aries." However, currently the vernal equinox is pointing toward the constellation Pisces.

The ECI reference frame is the simplest frame in which to describe a satellite's orbit because in this frame the orbit is a closed curve (an ellipse).

## 3.2 Earth Centered Fixed (ECF) Reference Frame

This reference frame rotates along with the Earth. The *x*-axis of the reference frame passes through the intersection of the Greenwich Meridian and the equator. The *z*-axis is the axis of Earth's rotation. Latitudes and longitudes are defined in the ECF reference frame; hence this frame is used for representing the location of a satellite in terms of geographic coordinates. More specifically, the ground trace of a satellite, i.e., the locus of points defined by the radial projection of the satellite on the Earth's surface, is defined in the ECF reference frame.

## 3.3 Topocentric Reference Frame

The topocentric reference frame is centered at an observer on the Earth. The $x$-axis points south, the $y$-axis due east, and the $z$-axis toward the observer's zenith, as shown in *Figure 6*. The topocentric coordinate frame is used in everyday life to give directions. In satellite geometry, the topocentric reference frame is used to describe the relative geometry between an observer and the satellite.

# 4. REFERENCE FRAME TRANSFORMATIONS

## 4.1 ECI to ECF

One of the prime uses of the ECI to ECF frame transformation is to determine the location of a satellite, or more accurately, the location of the sub-satellite point at a given instant of time in terms of latitude and longitude, with time usually expressed in the commonly used Gregorian calendar.

The transformation is from a reference frame stationary in space to a reference frame that rotates with the Earth. At a given instant of time, the ECF reference frame subtends an angle with the ECI reference frame. This angle, which is the angle between the vernal equinox and the Greenwich Meridian is called the Greenwich mean sidereal time, or GMST. Note that GMST is angle and not time. Also, GMST should not be confused with Greenwich Mean Time (GMT), which is the local time in London. To clarify this confusion, we use the term "GMST angle" instead of GMST.

It so happens that time expressed in the Gregorian calendar is not convenient to compute the GMST angle. It needs to be converted into a time-frame in which the computation of the GMST angle is simple. This time reference frame is the Julian time. Hence, the two steps involved in the computation of the GMST angle at a specific time instant are, (i) convert time from Gregorian calendar to Julian time, and (ii) determine the GMST angle subtended at the computed Julian time.

**1. Conversion to Julian time**

A few definitions first: "Universal Time" (UT) is the local time in the United Kingdom. The "Julian Day" (JD) is a continuous count of days and fractions thereof from noon on the first day of the year 4713 B.C. It is important to note that Julian Day starts at noon, i.e., $12^h$ UT.

The following is the algorithm to compute Julian day from Universal Time, from [3] pg. 60-61:

- Let Y represent the year, M the month (1 for January, 2 for February, etc., to 12 for December) and D the day of the month (with decimals, if any) of the given calendar date.
- If M > 2, leave Y and M unchanged.
  If M = 1 or 2, replace Y by Y-1 and M by M+12.
- Calculate:

$$A = \left\lfloor \frac{Y}{100} \right\rfloor \qquad\qquad B = 2 - A + \left\lfloor \frac{A}{4} \right\rfloor \tag{15}$$

- The required Julian Day is

$$JD = \lfloor 365.25(Y + 4716) \rfloor + \lfloor 30.6001(M + 1) \rfloor + D + B - 1524.5 \tag{16}$$

**2. GMST angle at a Julian time**

Again, from [3] pg. 87-88, the algorithm is:

- Find T by

$$T = \frac{JD - 2451545.0}{36525} \tag{17}$$

The GMST angle, in degrees, is given by

$$\begin{aligned} GMST = \; & 280.46061837 + 360.98564736629(JD - 2451545.0) \\ & + 0.000387933 \; T^2 - T^3 / 38710000 \end{aligned} \tag{18}$$

Now that we have computed the GMST angle at the specified time, we are set to convert from ECI to ECF reference frame. The transformation is a rotation about the *z*-axis by GMST angle. The transformation is efficiently computed using Cartesian coordinates. Let $(x,y,z)$ define the location of a point (say, a satellite) in the ECI reference frame and $(x',y',z')$ define the same coordinates in the ECF reference frame. The transformation, a rotation about the *z*-axis by angle –GMST, is given by

$$x' = x\cos GMST + y\sin GMST$$
$$y' = -x\sin GMST + y\cos GMST \tag{19}$$
$$z' = z$$

The longitude $\lambda_s$ and latitude $\phi_s$ of the point are given by

$$\tan\lambda_s = \frac{y'}{x'}$$
$$\tan\phi_s = \frac{z'}{\sqrt{x'^2 + y'^2}} \tag{20}$$

The length of the radial vector from the Earth's center to the point is given by

$$r = \sqrt{x'^2 + y'^2 + z'^2} = \sqrt{x^2 + y^2 + z^2} \tag{21}$$

## 4.2 ECF to Topocentric Frame

The topocentric reference frame is used to track a satellite in an arbitrary orbit from a point on the ground and usually requires the computation of quantities such as slant range, azimuth, and elevation. There are two approaches to computing these quantities, (i) using Cartesian geometry, and (ii) using spherical geometry.

### 4.2.1 Cartesian Geometry Based Transformation

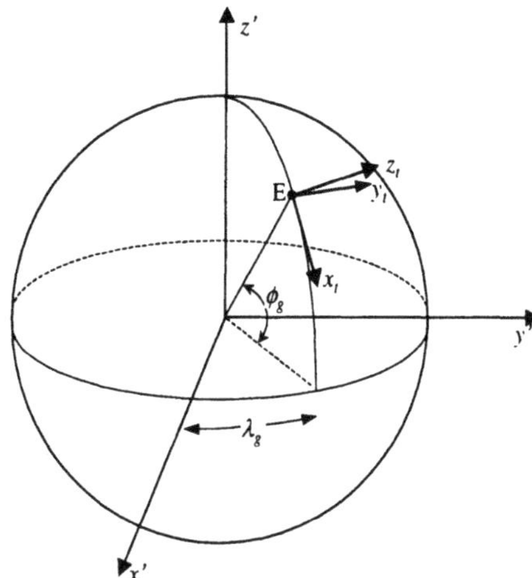


*Figure 6.* Earth-centered fixed coordinates and topocentric coordinates.

Let the Cartesian coordinates of the satellite in ECF coordinate frame be denoted by $(x',y',z')$ and the observer on the ground be located at longitude $\lambda_g$ and latitude $\phi_g$, as shown in *Figure 6*. The Cartesian coordinates of the observer in the ECF reference frame are

$$\begin{aligned} x'_g &= r_E \cos\phi_g \cos\lambda_g \\ y'_g &= r_E \cos\phi_g \sin\lambda_g \\ z'_g &= r_E \sin\phi_g \end{aligned} \tag{21}$$

The components of the slant range vector from the observer to the satellite are thus

$$\begin{bmatrix} \rho_x \\ \rho_y \\ \rho_z \end{bmatrix} = \begin{bmatrix} x' - x'_g \\ y' - y'_g \\ z' - z'_g \end{bmatrix} \tag{22}$$

For the transformation to topocentric coordinates $(x_t, y_t, z_t)$, we observe that topocentric coordinates involve (i) a rotation about the $z$ axis by angle $-\lambda_g$ followed by (ii) rotation about the $y$ axis by angle $-(90-\phi_g)$. Hence,

$$\begin{bmatrix} x_t \\ y_t \\ z_t \end{bmatrix} = \begin{bmatrix} \sin\phi_g & 0 & -\cos\phi_g \\ 0 & 1 & 0 \\ \cos\phi_g & 0 & \sin\phi_g \end{bmatrix} \begin{bmatrix} \cos\lambda_g & \sin\lambda_g & 0 \\ -\sin\lambda_g & \cos\lambda_g & 0 \\ 0 & 0 & 1 \end{bmatrix} \begin{bmatrix} \rho_x \\ \rho_y \\ \rho_z \end{bmatrix} \tag{23}$$

$$\begin{bmatrix} x_t \\ y_t \\ z_t \end{bmatrix} = \begin{bmatrix} \sin\phi_g \cos\lambda_g & \sin\phi_g \sin\lambda_g & -\cos\phi_g \\ -\sin\lambda_g & \cos\lambda_g & 0 \\ \cos\phi_g \cos\lambda_g & \cos\phi_g \sin\lambda_g & \sin\phi_g \end{bmatrix} \begin{bmatrix} \rho_x \\ \rho_y \\ \rho_z \end{bmatrix} \tag{24}$$

The slant range $d$ is

$$d = \sqrt{\rho_x^2 + \rho_y^2 + \rho_z^2} = \sqrt{x_t^2 + y_t^2 + z_t^2} \tag{25}$$

Also, the azimuth $Az$ and elevation angle $\theta$ are given by

$$\tan Az = \frac{y_t}{x_t} \tag{26}$$

and

$$\tan\theta = \frac{z_t}{\sqrt{x_t^2 + y_t^2}} \tag{27}$$

### 4.2.2 Spherical Geometry Based Transformation

The local mean sidereal time (LMST), again actually LMST angle, of a ground station at latitude $\lambda_g$, i.e., the angle between the vernal equinox and $\phi_g$ measured positive to the east, is LMST = GMST + $\lambda_g$.

The longitude of the satellite is given by

$$\lambda_s = \alpha - GMST \tag{28}$$

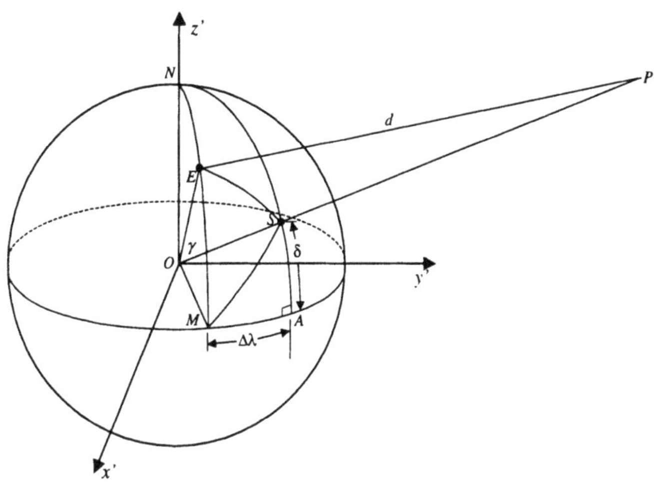


*Figure 7.* Geometry of a satellite with respect to an Earth station.

The geometry between the Earth station E and the satellite P with sub-satellite point S is shown in *Figure 7*. The hour angle $H$ of the satellite, measured positive to the west, is the relative longitude between $E$ and $S$, $H = -(\lambda_s - \lambda_g) \equiv -\Delta\lambda$. The spherical triangle *ENS* is redrawn in *Figure 8*. To compute the central angle $\gamma$ subtended by the great circle arc *ES*, we apply the law of cosines for sides to *ENS*

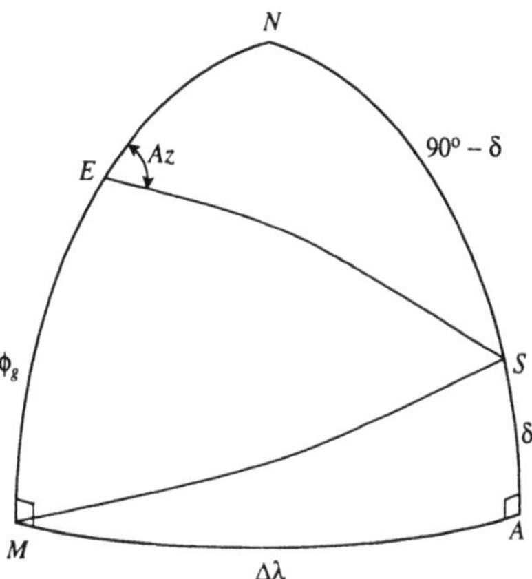


*Figure 8.* Spherical triangle *ENS*.

$$\cos\gamma = \cos(90-\delta)\cos(90-\phi_g) + \sin(90-\delta)\sin(90-\phi_g)\cos\Delta\lambda \\ = \sin\phi_g \sin\delta + \cos\phi_g \cos\delta\cos\Delta\lambda \tag{29}$$

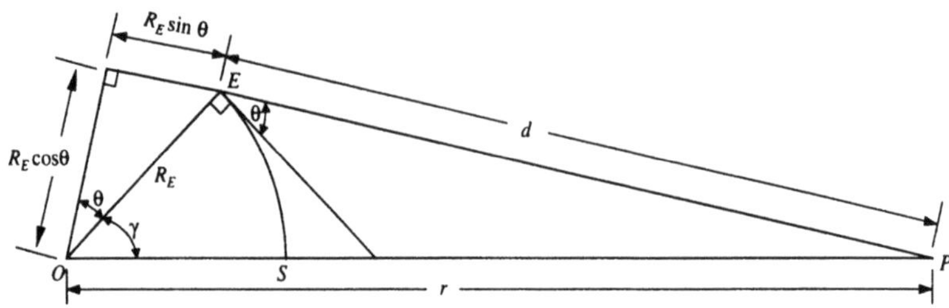


*Figure 9.* Plane triangle *EOP*.

The slant range $d$ is determined by the law of cosines applied to the plane triangle EOP, redrawn in *Figure 9*

$$d = \sqrt{R_E^2 + r^2 - 2R_E r\cos\gamma} \\ = \sqrt{R_E^2 + r^2 - 2R_E r(\sin\phi_g \sin\delta + \cos\phi_g \cos\delta\cos\Delta\lambda)} \tag{30}$$

The azimuth angle $Az$ is given by

$$\frac{\sin Az}{\sin(90-\delta)} = \frac{\sin\Delta\lambda}{\sin\gamma} \tag{31}$$

or

$$\sin Az = \frac{\cos\delta\sin\Delta\lambda}{\sin\gamma} \tag{32}$$

The elevation angle $\theta$ is obtained from the law of sines applied to plane triangle *EOP*

$$\frac{\sin(90+\theta)}{r} = \frac{\sin\gamma}{d} \tag{33}$$

or

$$\cos\theta = \frac{r}{d}\sin\gamma \tag{34}$$

# 5. PERTURBATION EFFECTS

As might be expected, perturbation effects differ in their significance for LEO satellites from that for satellites at much higher orbits. For example, the oblateness of the Earth affects LEO satellites to a greater degree than higher orbiting satellites and conversely the effects of the Sun's and Moon's gravity are more significant to higher orbiting satellites than for LEOs. The two important perturbations of the LEO orbits due to the Earth's oblateness are *nodal regression* and *apsidal precession*. The equations and a discussion is found in Wertz [5].

## 5.1 Nodal Regression

The line that is common to the equatorial plane and the orbital plane is called the *line of nodes*. This line precesses at a rate that is dependent upon the magnitude of the satellite orbit's semi-major axis ($a$ is in kilometers), eccentricity, and inclination. The rate of precession is approximately $-2.06474 \cdot 10^{14} \cdot a^{-7/2} \cdot (1-e^2)^{-2} \cdot \cos i$ degrees per day. If the rate of precession is 0.9856 degrees per day, then we have the interesting case wherein the line of nodes turns around $360^0$ in one year. The effect of this specific rate is that the satellite's orbital plane remains essentially fixed with respect to the sun and also views the Earth below at the same angle. Such an orbit is called *sun synchronous*. (Note that a sun synchronous orbit is retrograde as $\cos i$ must be negative.) In *Figure 10* we plot the inclination, $i$, in degrees, versus the apogee height of a circular orbit in order that the satellite orbit be sun synchronous.

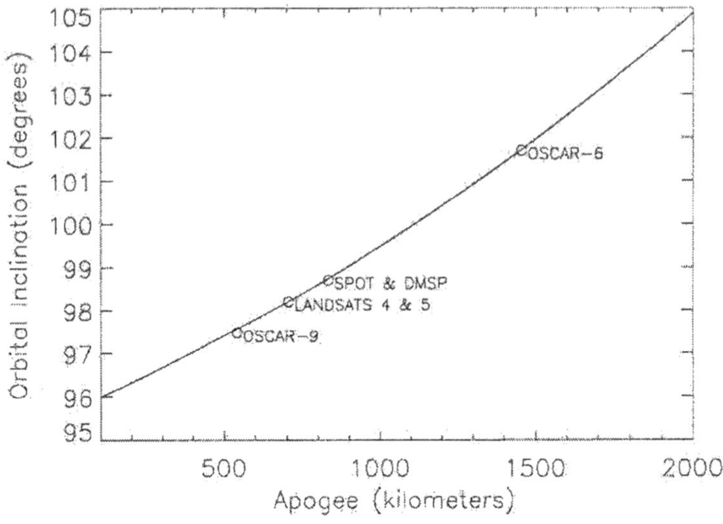


*Figure 10.* Inclination required for a circular satellite orbit to be sun synchronous.

## 5.2 Apsidal Precession

Another line of importance is the line that passes through the satellite's position at perigee and apogee. This line is called the *line of apsides* and it also precesses due to an orbital perturbation. The rate of precession is approximately $2.06474 \cdot 10^{14} \cdot a^{-7/2} \cdot (1-e^2)^{-2} \cdot (2-\frac{5}{2}\sin^2 i)$, again with $a$ in kilometers. This perturbation is not important, of course, if we are dealing with circular orbits.

The most striking example of the implications of this perturbation, incidentally, is found in the design of the so-called Molniya orbit. The Molniya orbit was the orbit chosen for a class of satellites that served the massive landmass of the former USSR. The orbits were highly elliptical with the apogee over the Northern Hemisphere. Having the apogee there allowed the satellites to spend a great proportion of their orbital period in common view of the USSR ground stations served. Clearly the converse situation, an exchange of apogee and perigee, would be of little utility. There was thus a desire to keep the apsidal precession negligible and this was achieved by correctly setting the inclination, $i$. The Molniya orbit was inclined at about $i = 63.4^o$ and this caused the multiplicative term, $(2-\frac{5}{2}\sin^2 i)$, to vanish, thus nullifying the apsidal precession.

Another important consideration is atmospheric drag. The LEO orbit, as it is so near to the Earth, will encounter traces of atmosphere that will act on the satellite and eventually cause orbital decay. Key parameters for calculating estimated time of terminal orbital decay are initial perigee, eccentricity, satellite mass, and satellite cross-sectional geometry. For this last variable, it is important to know the area presented to the vestigial atmosphere. The greater the area, the more decelerating momentum transfer there will be, and the sooner the satellite will decay.

*Figure 11* is a graphical aid from [6]. It is useful for making a crude estimate of time to terminal orbital decay. Aside from knowing the relevant satellite orbital elements, we are required to know or estimate the satellite's *ballistic coefficient* in order to use *Figure 11*. The ballistic coefficient is defined as $\frac{m}{C_D A}$ where $m$ is the satellite's mass, $A$ is the satellite's cross-sectional area normal to the direction of the satellite's motion, and $C_D$ is the drag coefficient. Wertz [5] suggests that, if unknown, $C_D$ be picked in the range from 1 to 2. Wertz [5] cautions that "Most lifetime estimates are in error by at least 10%. Simplified relations ... [such as *Figure 11*] may be in error by 50%."

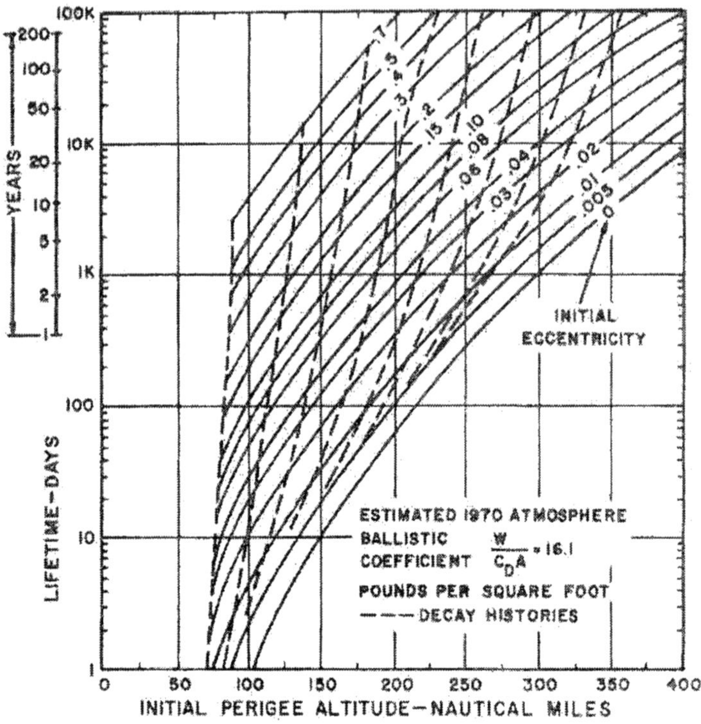


*Figure 11.* Lifetime due to atmospheric drag.

In order to gain a perspective on LEO orbital decay times, we have compiled Table 3 from the SSTL database [2]. Table 3 is a selection of some crucial parameters of LEO satellites that have decayed.

*Table 3.* Some LEO satellites that have undergone terminal orbital decay.

| Satellite Name | Date of Launch | Date of Decay | Lifetime (days) | Mass (kg) | Orbit (km x km) | Inclination (deg) | Shape |
|---|---|---|---|---|---|---|---|
| Rahini-2 | 5/31/81 | 6/8/81 | 8 | 38 | 186x418 | 46.27 | Spherical 0.6 m (diam.) |
| OSCAR -2 | 6/2/62 | 6/21/62 | 19 | - | 384x206 | 73 | - |
| Iskra-3 | 11/18/82 | 12/16/82 | 28 | 28 | 345x346 | 51.63 | Spherical 0.6 m (diam.) |
| OSCAR -1 | 12/12/61 | 1/31/62 | 50 | 4.5 | 372x211 | 81 | - |
| Iskra-2 | 5/17/82 | 7/9/82 | 53 | 28 | 335x345 | 51.59 | Spherical 0.6 m (diam.) |
| ESRO-I (BOREA) | 10/1/69 | 11/23/69 | 53 | 86? | 393x306 | 85.12 | Cylindrical 760 mm (diam.) 930 mm (height) |
| Sputnik-I | 10/4/57 | 1/4/58 | 92 | 83.6 | 215x939 | 65.1 | Spherical 0.58 m (diam.) |
| MicroSats | 7/16/91 | 1/23-25/92 | ~192 | 22 | 359x457 | 82 | - |
| San Marco-1 | 12/15/64 | 9/13/65 | 272 | 24 | 194x697 | 38 | - |
| BREMSAT | 2/94 | 2/12/95 | ~363 | 63 | 363x344 | 56.0 | - |
| ESRO-I (AURORAE) | 10/3/68 | 6/26/70 | 631 | 86 | 1534x254 | 93.76 | Cylindrical 760 mm (diam.) 930 mm (height) |
| GLOMR | 10/26/85 | ~2/26/85 | ~420 | 68 | 326 | 57 | Spherical 0.25 m (diam.) |
| ESRO-II (IRIS) | 5/17/68 | 5/9/71 | 1087 | 75 | 1094x332 | 97.21 | Cylindrical 760 mm (diam.) 850 mm (height) |
| Ariel-3 | 5/5/67 | Dec/70 | ~1320 | 90 | 498x606 | 80 | - |
| Ariel-2 | 3/27/64 | 12/18/67 | 1361 | 68 | 285x1362 | 52 | - |
| Losat-X | 7/4/91 | 11/15/95 | 1595 | 75 | 416x402 | 40 | 1.2 m x 0.9 m x 0.3 m |
| MIKA | 3/10/70 | 9/9/74 | 1644 | 52 | 1746x307 | 5 | - |
| Taiyo | 2/24/75 | 6/29/80 | 1952 | 86 | 255x3135 | 31 | - |
| Hakucho (Corsa-B) | 2/21/79 | 4/15/85 | 2245 | 96 | 541x572 | 29.9 | Prism 650 mm x 800 MM |

Consider the two satellites Iskra-3 and GLOMR. We first calculate the ballistic coefficients for these two satellites. They are both spherical and so calculating the satellite's cross-sectional area normal to the direction of the satellite's motion is straightforward. If we assume $C_D = 1.5$, we have the data shown in Table 4.

*Table 4*. Terminal decay data for two spherical LEO satellites.

| Satellite | Initial Perigee (n miles) | Ballistic Coefficient (lb per square foot) | Predicted Time to Terminal Decay (days) | Actual Time to Terminal Decay (days) |
|---|---|---|---|---|
| Iskra-3 | 186.6 | 13.5 | 33 | 28 |
| GLOMR | 176 | 189 | 352 | 420 |

# 6. THE UPLINK INTERFERENCE ENVIRONMENT

It is important to estimate the interference environment experienced at the satellite's uplink receiver(s). A few studies have been performed in which the interference was mapped across the globe. A summary of one of these important studies, Paffett et al. [7], advises that "The frequency bands allocated by the WARC92 for use by 'Little LEO' systems are still shared with terrestrial services, and it is shown using results from the in-orbit measurements that the interference in these bands can severely limit the performance of a narrow band satellite communication system. One can consider usage of these frequencies by other users, be it terrestrial or satellite, as a form of interference, which must be accommodated for successful system operations." The study involved the monitoring of two adjacent 25-kHz channels within the 148–150 MHz uplink band. The satellite platform was the HealthSat II Little LEO, which had a circular orbit of 800-km height and was in near polar orbit with an inclination of 89.5 degrees.

*Figure 12* displays the mean received signal strength observed in two adjacent 25 kHz channels and Figure 13 displays the dynamic range of the observed received signal strengths. The range of signal power in *Figure 12* is on the order of 50 dB. The lighter areas represent higher levels of interference. It is perhaps not that surprising that the heavily industrialized areas show the highest interference levels. In *Figure 13*, the regions exhibiting large variations in received signal strength are colored more darkly. These figures are provided courtesy of J. Paffett and colleagues, Surrey Space Centre, Surrey University, and reproduced with permission.

So important and so potentially deleterious is the uplink interference environment that special and sophisticated measures may be required for some communication systems. The proposed STARSYS system [8], intended to "provide commercial messaging and localization services between mobile terminals and regional stations, connected to processing facilities and user's networks," is said to employ a "proprietary interference rejection processing, using frequency domain adaptive filtering" in order to excise significant narrowband jammers.

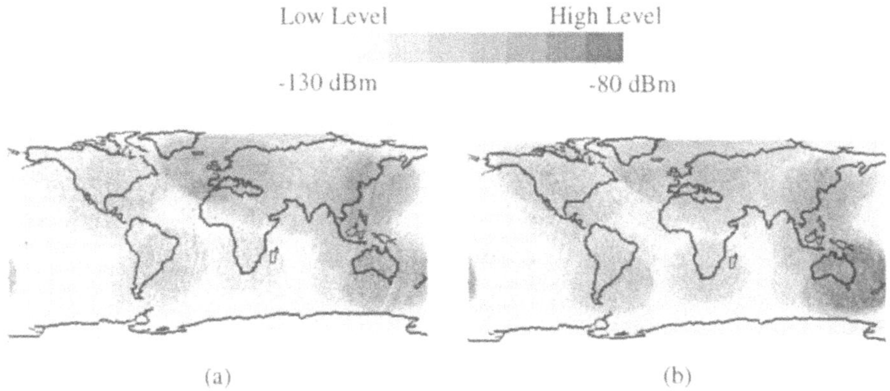


*Figure 12.* Mean received signal strength in two 25 kHz channels.

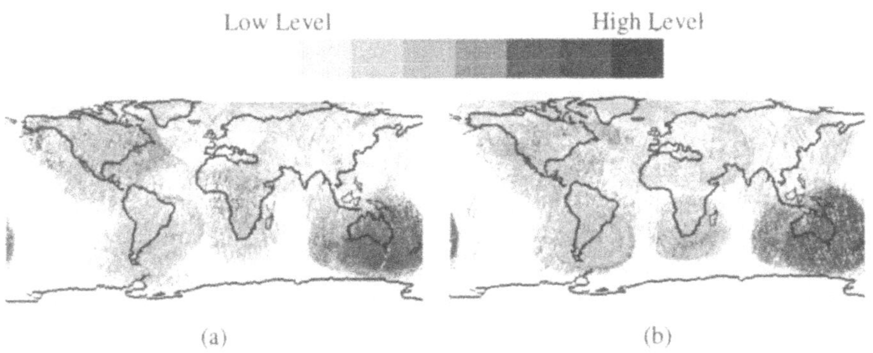


*Figure 13.* Dynamic range of the observed received signal strength in two 25-kHz channels.

## REFERENCES

[1] M. Sturza, "LEOs-the communications satellites of the 21st century," Northcon/96 Proceedings, pp. 114-118, 1996.

[2] SSTL (Surrey Space Centre, Surrey University) Web published data on LEO satellites.

[3] J. Meeus, Astronomical Algorithms, Second Edition, Willmann-Bell Inc., 1998.

[4] http://oig1.gsfc.nasa.gov. NASA's web site for orbit parameters of satellites.

[5]Spacecraft Attitude Determination and Control, James Wertz , Ed., D. Reidel Publishing Company, 1978

[6] Space Planners Guide, United States Air Force, Air Force Systems Command, 1 July 1965,.

[7] Paffett, J., da Silva Curiel, R., Jeans, T., Ward, J., and M. Sweeting, "In-orbit measurement and analysis of the 'Little-LEO' VHF uplink frequencies using a LEO microsatellite," GLOBECOM'97, Vol. 2, pp. 1138-1141, 1997.

[8] Serene, B., Collomby, M., Dribault, L., and E. Beaufume, "The STARSYS System and Satellite Concept to Provide World-Wide Commercial Services Including Two-Way Messaging and Localisation," Space Technology, Vol. 17, No. 1, pp. 51-57, 1997.

Chapter 2

# Doppler Characterization

In this chapter, we derive an equation for Doppler-time curves at ground based terminals on the forward channel due to the relative motion of a circular orbit LEO satellite. We show that Doppler-time curves can be classified based solely on the maximum elevation angle between the terminal and satellite during the satellite's visibility window. This characterization depends only on the relative geometry between the terminal and the satellite. We also derive an expression for the visibility window duration of the satellite as a function of the maximum elevation angle. We then provide an algorithm for estimating the parameters of a Doppler curve based on a pair of Doppler and Doppler-rate measurements.

## 1. INTRODUCTION

For satellite communications through LEO satellites, mobile units (terminals) or Earth stations observe significant Doppler, which has to be estimated and compensated for, to enable reliable communication. In this chapter we mathematically characterize the Doppler shift observed at points on Earth for circular orbit satellites.

We also introduce an algorithm that can be used by mobile terminals to predict, at the onset of satellite visibility, the shape of the Doppler-time variation over the remainder of the visibility duration. The Doppler curve information may be used to improve the performance of the terminal's phase-locked-loop. Moreover, the terminal can also estimate the duration of the visibility window and the instant of maximum elevation. This could be used as a basis for multiple access by scheduling transmission of packets from the terminal at higher elevation angles to the satellite. A more elaborate multiple-access scheme based on Doppler characterization has been proposed in [4] and is covered in Chapter 5. The Doppler characterization can be used to predict the visibility-time function of a satellite at a terminal; this was proposed in [5] and is covered in Chapter 4. Effective power conservation at the terminal, by switching the power supply off during the non-visibility periods and then switching it on based on the visibility-time information, can also be implemented.

Previous research has primarily focused on methodology to compensate for Doppler shifts. Only in [1,2] did the authors attempt to characterize Doppler-time curves. In [1] the authors considered the simple case of circular LEO satellites in the equatorial plane and Doppler observed by points on the equator. However, they did not consider the general case of inclined circular orbits and points not on the ground trace. In [2] the authors derived expressions for the time-evolution of elevation angle and Doppler for elliptical orbit satellites. However, they did not parameterize Doppler curves observed by points on Earth.

## 2. DOPPLER CURVE

For LEO satellites, the Doppler frequency at terminals exhibits well-behaved variation with time that can be parameterized by the maximum elevation angle from the terminal to the satellite during the visibility window. This S shaped variation is depicted in *Figure 14* for maximum elevation angles ranging from $11.4^0$ to $90^0$ degrees for a terminal located at latitude $39^0$ *N* and longitude $77^0$ *W*. The satellite follows a circular orbit (eccentricity=0) of altitude 1000 km and inclination $53^0$. The minimum elevation angle for visibility is assumed to be $10^0$. Doppler shift is captured in terms of normalized Doppler shift which is equal to $(v/c)$, where $v$ is the relative velocity of the satellite with respect to the terminal and $c$ is the speed of light. Time is expressed relative to the zero-Doppler instant. The zero-Doppler instant is the time during the visibility window at which the elevation angle from the terminal to the satellite is at its maximum value and the satellite is at its closest approach to the terminal. The Doppler frequency shift is shown only for the visibility duration of the satellite at the terminal; the visibility duration increases as the maximum elevation angle to the satellite increases.

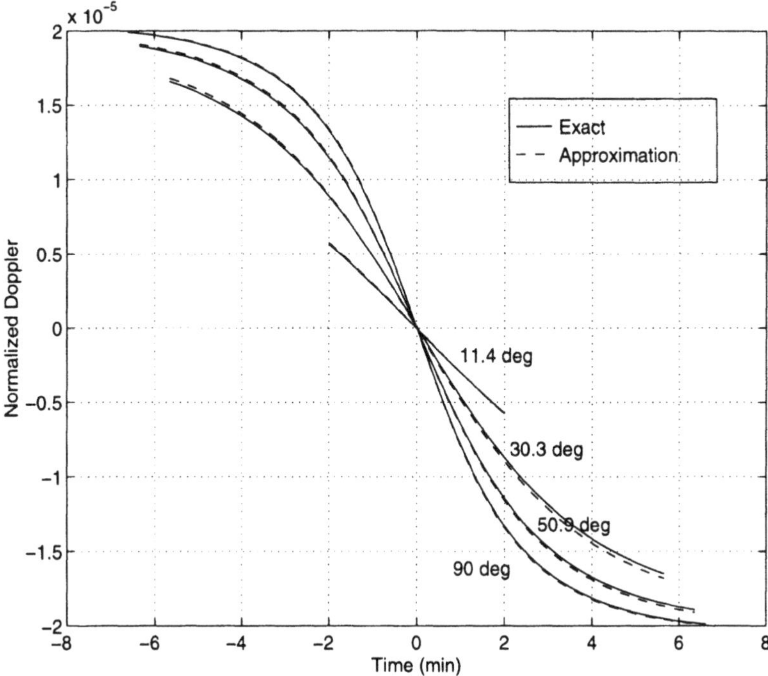


*Figure 14.* Actual and approximate Doppler S-curve for different maximum elevation angles.

## 2.1 Analysis Strategy

The first step in our analysis is to derive from geometry, the equation for the observed Doppler shift for a given terminal location and a maximum elevation angle. The analysis is performed as seen from the terminal's location, i.e., in the Earth-centered fixed (ECF) coordinate frame, using trigonometric formulas for spherical triangles. To use the spherical triangle laws, we make the assumption that in the ECF frame the satellite's orbit during the visibility window can be approximated by a great-circle arc. We then show that the variation in the angular velocity of the satellite in the ECF frame is very small (<3%) for most LEO circular orbits and hence, can be approximated by a constant. We next derive the equation for the visibility window duration of a satellite for a given maximum elevation angle.

## 2.2 Doppler Equation

Consider the geometry of *Figure 15*. The coordinate system is an ECF coordinate system. Point *P* denotes the location of the terminal, which observes a maximum elevation angle $\theta_{max}$. A segment of the ground along with the segment of the satellite's orbit trace is shown. Point $M$ is the sub-satellite point at the instant the terminal observes maximum elevation angle.

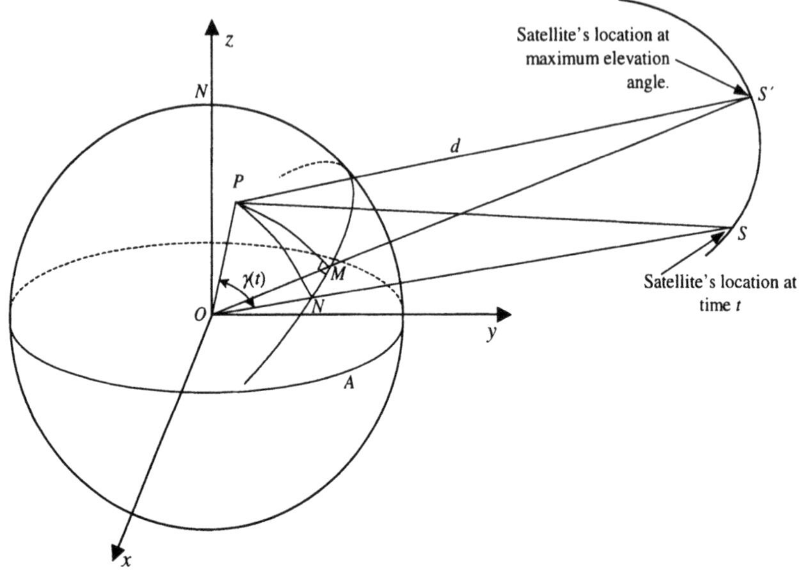


*Figure 15.* Satellite geometry during visibility window at location $P$.

In the ECF frame the satellite's orbit is not a great circle due to the rotation of the Earth (see [3], Figure 2-15, pp. 72). However, the visibility window at a point on Earth for a LEO satellite is small compared to the orbit period. For example, for a circular orbit altitude of 1000 km, the maximum visibility window duration is less than 14 minutes whereas the orbit period is 1.75 hours. Hence, for the visibility window duration the deviation of the satellite's orbit from a great-circle arc is small.

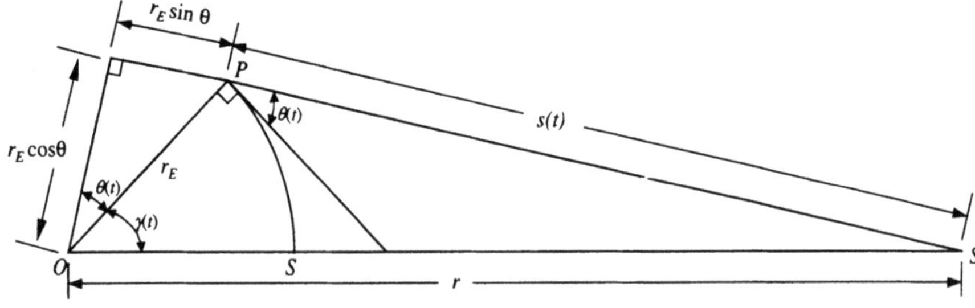


*Figure 16.* Plane triangle *SOP*.

The slant range $s(t)$ is determined by the law of cosines applied to the plane triangle *SOP*, redrawn in *Figure 16*,

$$s(t) = \sqrt{r_E^2 + r^2 - 2r_E r \cos\gamma(t)} \qquad (1)$$

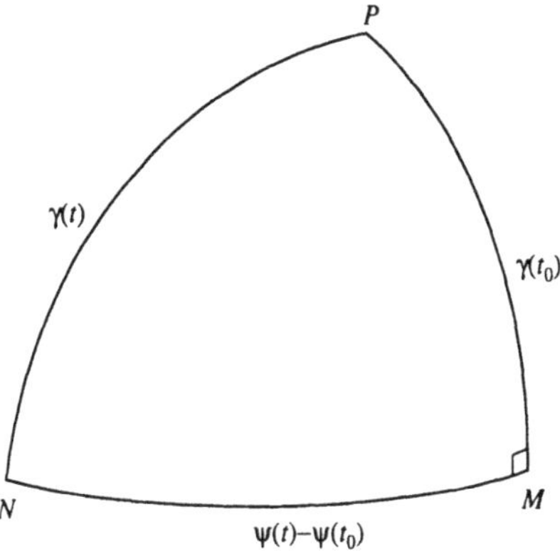


*Figure 17.* Spherical triangle *MNP*.

Let $t_0$ denote the instant when the terminal observes maximum elevation angle and $\psi - \psi(t_0)$ is the angular distance between *M* and *N* measured on the surface of Earth along the ground trace. From the cosine law of sides applied to the spherical right triangle *MNP* (*Figure 17*),

$$\cos\gamma(t) = \cos(\psi(t) - \psi(t_0))\cos\gamma(t_0) \qquad (2)$$

Differentiating the above expression and substituting it into the expression for the derivative of the slant range, we have

$$\dot{s}(t) = \frac{r_E r \sin(\psi(t) - \psi(t_0))\cos\gamma(t_0) \cdot \dot{\psi}(t)}{\sqrt{r_E^2 + r^2 - 2r_E r\cos(\psi(t) - \psi(t_0))\cos\gamma(t_0)}} \qquad (3)$$

Also, from *Figure 16*, the central angle at epoch of maximum elevation angle, $\theta(t_0) = \theta_{\max}$, satisfies

$$\cos(\theta_{\max} + \gamma(t_0)) = \frac{r_E}{r}\cos\theta_{\max} \qquad (4)$$

Now $\dot{\psi}(t)$ is the angular velocity of the satellite in the ECF frame, which we shall denote as $\omega_F(t)$. Substituting $\dot{\psi}(t) = \omega_F(t)$ in Equation (3) and noting that normalized Doppler $(\Delta f / f)$ is given by $-\dot{s}(t)/c$ where $c$ is the speed of light, we obtain,

$$\frac{\Delta f}{f} = -\frac{1}{c}\frac{r_E r \sin(\psi(t)-\psi(t_0))\cos\left(\cos^{-1}\left(\frac{r_E}{r}\cos\theta_{\max}\right)-\theta_{\max}\right)\cdot\omega_F(t)}{\sqrt{r_E^2 + r^2 - 2r_E r\cos(\psi(t)-\psi(t_0))\cos\left(\cos^{-1}\left(\frac{r_E}{r}\cos\theta_{\max}\right)-\theta_{\max}\right)}} \quad (5)$$

From the above expression, we observe that the normalized Doppler is a function of the maximum elevation angle $\theta_{max}$ and the angular velocity $\omega_F(t)$ of the satellite in the ECF frame.

## 2.3 Satellite Velocity

In the Earth-centered inertial (ECI) frame the angular velocity is constant; however, in the ECF frame it varies with latitude due to Earth's rotation.

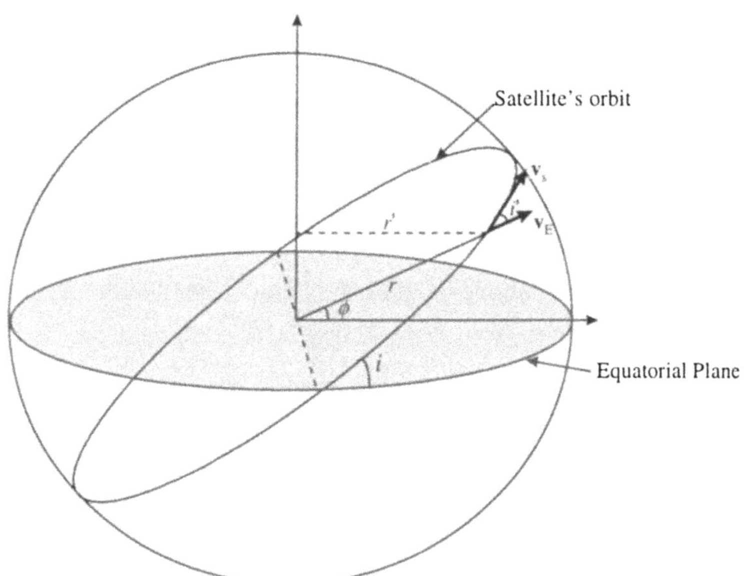


*Figure 18.* Satellite's tangential velocity in the ECI frame.

Consider the geometry of *Figure 18*. Let $i$ denote the inclination of the orbit. The angular velocity of the satellite in the ECI coordinate system is denoted by $\omega_s$. The corresponding tangential velocity of the satellite in the ECI frame is denoted by $\vec{\mathbf{v}}_s$. Vector $\vec{\mathbf{v}}_E(\phi)$ denotes the velocity of the sub-satellite point due to Earth's rotation at latitude $\phi$ degrees projected up to the satellite's altitude. Vector $\vec{\mathbf{v}}_F(\phi)$ (not shown in the figure) denotes the corresponding velocity of the satellite in the ECF frame, and is given by the resultant

$$\vec{\mathbf{v}}_F(\phi) = \vec{\mathbf{v}}_s - \vec{\mathbf{v}}_E(\phi) \tag{6}$$

Using the triangle law of cosines and the relation $\cos i' = \cos i / \cos\phi$, and letting $\omega_E$ denote the angular velocity of the Earth's rotation,

$$|v_F(\phi)|^2 = |v_s|^2 + r^2\omega_E^2\cos^2\phi - 2r\ \omega_E|v_s|\cos i \tag{7}$$

Numerically, for LEO satellites, the absolute variation of the satellite's velocity in the ECF frame for a given orbit is very small. For an orbit of inclination $i = 60^0$ and altitude $h$ = 500km, $|\mathbf{v}_F(0)|$ = 7.3747km/s and $|\mathbf{v}_F(60^0)|$ = 7.3619km/s. The percentage variation of $|\mathbf{v}_F|$ with respect to $|\mathbf{v}_s|$ (i.e., $\Delta|\mathbf{v}_F|/|\mathbf{v}_s|$) is only 0.168 %. For orbit altitude $h$=2000km, the variation is 0.3073%, and for $h$ = 10,000km, it is 2.466%. Hence, for low to medium orbit altitudes, the magnitude of the tangential velocity of the satellite in the ECF frame shows small variation, and can be approximated by a constant. We approximate $|\mathbf{v}_F(\phi)|$ by its value at the highest latitude, i.e.,

$$|v_F| \approx |v_s| - r\omega_E\cos i \tag{8}$$

Therefore,

$$\omega_F \approx \omega_s - \omega_E\cos i \tag{9}$$

We should note here that $|v_F(\varphi)| \geq |v_F(\iota)|, \nabla\varphi$. Hence, we have approximated $|v_F(\phi)|$ by its minimum value.

## 2.4 Satellite Visibility Window Duration

Let $t_v$ denote the time when the satellite just becomes visible to the terminal. The angle of elevation to the satellite at $t_v$, denoted $\theta_v$, is the minimum elevation angle for visibility.

From the cosine law of sides applied to the right triangle *NMP* (*Figure 17*),

$$\cos\gamma(t_v) = \cos\big(\psi(t_v) - \psi(t_0)\big)\cos\gamma(t_0) \tag{10}$$

which implies

$$\psi(t_v) - \psi(t_0) = \omega_F(t_v - t_0) = \cos^{-1}\left(\frac{\cos\gamma(t_v)}{\cos\gamma(t_0)}\right) \tag{11}$$

Using the angular velocity approximation, and noting that the total visibility window duration of the satellite at the terminal, $\tau(\theta_{max})$, is $2|t_v - t_0|$, we have

$$\tau(\theta_{max}) \approx \frac{2}{\omega_s - \omega_E \cos i}\cos^{-1}\left(\frac{\cos\left(\cos^{-1}\left(\frac{r_E}{r}\cos\theta_v\right) - \theta_v\right)}{\cos\left(\cos^{-1}\left(\frac{r_E}{r}\cos\theta_{max}\right) - \theta_{max}\right)}\right) \tag{12}$$

## 3. NUMERICAL RESULTS

The configuration for the numerical results consists of a satellite in a circular orbit (eccentricity=0) of altitude 1000 km and orbit inclination of $53^0$. The terminal is assumed to be located at $39^0$ *N* and $77^0$ *W* (Washington, D.C.). A computer orbit generation program was used to generate exact Doppler-time curves.

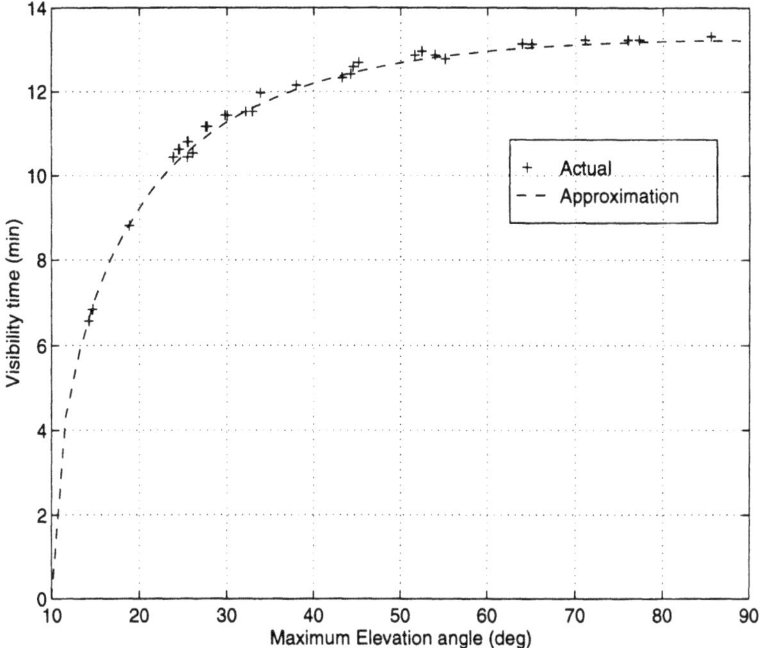


*Figure 19.* Actual and approximate satellite visibility window duration.

*Figure 14* consists of plots of exact normalized Doppler-time and the analytic Doppler-time (Equation (5)) approximation for a range of maximum elevation angles. In *Figure 19,* we provide numerical results for the visibility window duration versus maximum elevation angle. In *Figure 20* we plot results of the approximation error, in terms of coefficient of determination [6, pg. 449], between the Doppler-time approximation and the exact Doppler-time curves. The coefficient of determination, $R^2$, is defined as

$$R^2 = \frac{SS_{dd} - SSE}{SS_{dd}} \tag{13}$$

where $SS_{dd} = \sum (d_i - \bar{d})^2$ and $SSE = \sum (d_i - \hat{d}_i)^2$, with $\{d_i\}$ denoting data points for actual Doppler and $\{\hat{d}_i\}$ those for estimated Doppler.

We consider three orbit altitudes of 1000 km, 5000 km, and 10,000 km. The orbit inclination is $53^0$ in all three cases. The analytic approximations are excellent fits to the exact Doppler-time curves. We observe that the approximation error increases as the altitude of the orbit increases due to larger variations in the satellite's ECF velocity, as discussed in Section 2.3.

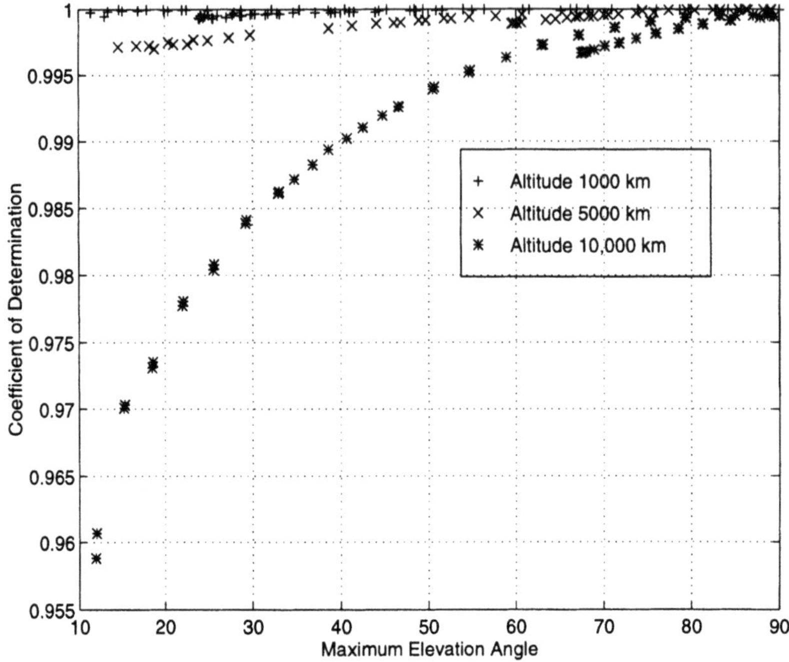


*Figure 20.* Accuracy of the Doppler-time approximation as a function of the maximum elevation angle for different orbit altitudes.

# 4. DOPPLER CURVE ESTIMATION

In this section, we show how to process Doppler and Doppler-rate measurements to compute estimates of the zero-Doppler time $t_0$ and the associated maximum elevation angle $\theta_{max}$.

Denoting the right-hand side of Equation (5) by $d(t)$, differentiating and manipulating the resulting expression, it can be shown that

$$\frac{r_E r \omega_F^2}{d^2(t)}\left(\frac{\sin\alpha(t)\dot{d}(t)}{\omega_F d(t)} - \cos\alpha(t)\right) = \frac{1}{\cos\gamma(t_0)} \tag{14}$$

where $\alpha(t) = \omega_F(t - t_0)$. Since the right side of Equation (14) is independent of time

$$\frac{r_E r \omega_F^2}{d_1^2}\left(\frac{\sin\alpha_1 \dot{d}_1}{\omega_F d_1} - \cos\alpha_1\right) = \frac{r_E r \omega_F^2}{d_2^2}\left(\frac{\sin\alpha_2 \dot{d}_2}{\omega_F d_2} - \cos\alpha_2\right) \tag{15}$$

where the subscripts 1 and 2 denote measurements made at sampling instants $t_1$ and $t_2$ ($>t_1$), respectively. Since $\alpha_1$ and $\alpha_2$ are related by $\alpha_2 = \alpha_1 + \omega_F (t_2 - t_1) = \alpha_1 + \omega_F \Delta t$, we can rewrite Equation (14) as follows

$$K_1 = \frac{\dot{d}_1}{\omega_F d_1}; \qquad K_2 = \frac{d_1^2 \dot{d}_2}{d_2^3 \omega_F}; \qquad K_3 = \frac{d_1^2}{d_2^2} \tag{16}$$

Using the trigonometric identities for sin($A$+$B$) and cos($A$+$B$), it can be readily shown that

$$\alpha_1 = \tan^{-1}\left( \frac{1 + K_2 \sin \omega_F \Delta t - K_3 \cos \omega_F \Delta t}{K_1 - K_2 \cos \omega_F \Delta t - K_3 \sin \omega_F \Delta t} \right) \tag{17}$$

The zero-Doppler time is computed from the relation

$$t_0 = t_1 - \frac{\alpha_1}{\omega_F} \tag{18}$$

From Equation (4), we have

$$\tan \theta_{\max} = \frac{\cos \gamma(t_0) - \frac{r_E}{r}}{\sin \gamma(t_0)} \tag{19}$$

where $\cos \gamma(t_0)$ is computed from Equation (4) and $\sin \gamma(t_0) = \pm\sqrt{1 - \cos^2 \gamma(t_0)}$ (since $0^0 \le \theta_{\max} \le 90^0$, one sign is rejected based on physical considerations).

## REFERENCES

[1] M. Katayama, A. Ogawa, and N. Morinaga, "Carrier Synchronization Under Doppler Shift of the Nongeostationary satellite communication system," *Proc. of ICCS/ISITA '92*, 1992, p. 466-470.

[2] E. Vilar and J. Austin, "Analysis and correction techniques of Doppler shift for non-geosynchronous communication satellites," *International Journal of Satellite Communications*, Vol. 9, 1991, p. 123-136.

[3] W.L. Pritchard, H.G. Suyderhoud and R.A. Nelson, *Satellite Communication Systems Engineering*, Prentice Hall, 1993.

[4] I. Ali, N. Al-Dhahir, J.E. Hershey, G.J. Saulnier, and R. Nelson, "Doppler as a New Dimension for Multiple-access in LEO Satellite Systems," *International Journal of Satellite Communications*, Vol. 15 No. 6, Nov-Dec 1997, p. 269-279.

[5] I. Ali, N. Al-Dhahir, and J.E. Hershey, "Predicting the Visibility of LEO Satellites," *IEEE Transactions on Aerospace and Electronic Systems,* Vol. 35, No. 4, October 1999, p. 1183-1189.

[6] W. Mendenhall and T. Sincich, *Statistics for Engineering and Computer Sciences*, Second Edition, Dellen Publishing Company, 1988.

# Chapter 3

# Doppler Estimation at Terminals

In this chapter we provide an overview of various open-loop frequency and phase estimation techniques suitable for packet-based LEO satellite communications. The Cramer-Rao lower bound on the variance of Doppler frequency and phase estimation is presented and is shown to decrease as $1/N^3$ and $1/N$, respectively, where $N$ is the number of processed discrete-time observations. This motivates the estimation of Doppler frequency before phase due to its faster convergence. While the maximum likelihood frequency estimator is theoretically optimum, it requires exhaustive search procedures that can be prohibitive in terms of computation and storage requirements. Alternatively, lower-complexity algorithms that average windowed estimates of the angle of several correlation lags of the discrete-time observations are presented. After the Doppler frequency is estimated accurately, its effect may be removed by de-rotating the received data symbols. Prior to data demodulation, an accurate estimate of any unknown phase offset may be calculated as the arctangent of the ratio of averaged quadrature to in-phase values of the de-rotated data symbols. Simulation results illustrate the effectiveness of the Doppler frequency estimation algorithms.

## 1. INTRODUCTION

The relative movement, whether approach or escape, of a LEO satellite with respect to a receiving terminal on the surface of the Earth causes a shift in the carrier frequency of the received satellite signal. This phenomenon is commonly referred to as the Doppler effect. In addition to frequency offsets which result in a *rotation* of the received signal constellation, random but fixed (over a data block) phase offsets are also common in packet-based data communications [9] and cause a *tilt* in the received signal constellation. Both effects can significantly degrade the quality of a satellite link unless they are accurately estimated and compensated for.

As will become clear in the ensuing chapters, the main theme of this book is that while the presence of a Doppler frequency shift impairs the quality of the received satellite signal if left uncompensated for, it also contains valuable information on the maximum elevation angle of a LEO satellite at a ground terminal. This information can be used at the ground terminals to enhance overall system performance.

Doppler frequency and phase estimation techniques can be broadly divided into two categories:

- *Closed-loop techniques,* such as those using a phase-locked loop (PLL) or decision-directed techniques. For short packet communications, PLLs cannot provide rapid acquisition of the carrier frequency and phase due to the hang-up phenomenon [5]. In addition, decision-directed frequency and phase techniques [2] are plagued with the effects of decision errors, which become more pronounced at low SNR levels where many LEO satellite links operate.
- *Open-loop techniques,* which operate on the in-phase and quadrature components of the digitized received signal without requiring feedback or the use of numerically or voltage-controlled oscillators. Furthermore, these techniques are derived from the maximum likelihood estimate under various assumptions and approximations, and are suitable for digital implementation. Therefore, we shall focus on open-loop techniques for the remainder of this chapter.

## 2. CRAMER-RAO LOWER BOUND

We start with the standard baseband model of a received data packet of length $N$ corrupted by additive white Gaussian noise, Doppler frequency $w_d$, and a random phase error $\theta$

$$r_k = x_k e^{j(w_d kT+\theta)} + n_k \quad k = 0,1,..,N-1 \tag{1}$$

where T is the symbol period.

For simplicity, we assume Binary Phase Shift Keying (BPSK) modulated data, i.e, $x_k \in \{\pm 1\}$. It is straightforward to extend the analysis to other modulation schemes.

The first step is to remove modulation effects from the received data. For BPSK modulation, this can be done by squaring[1] the received digitized samples. The squared samples have the form

$$z_k \overset{def}{=} r_k^{\ 2} \approx e^{j2(w_d kT+\theta)} + v_k \overset{def}{=} e^{j(w_0 k+\theta_0)} + v_k,\ k=0,1,..,N-1 \tag{2}$$

where $v_k$ is a noise sequence assumed to be zero-mean, Gaussian-distributed, and uncorrelated, with a variance equal to $\sigma_v^2$. Using the observations vector $\mathbf{z} \overset{def}{=} [z_0, z_1, \cdots, z_{N-1}]$, we would like to estimate the unknown vector $\mathbf{u} \overset{def}{=} [\theta_0, w_0]$, where $\theta_0 = 2\theta$ and $w_0 = 2w_d T$.

The conditional probability density function (pdf) of **z** given **u** is

$$p(z \mid \mathbf{u}) = F(\mathbf{z}) \exp(\frac{2}{\sigma_v^{\ 2}} \sum_{k=1}^{N} \Re(z_k e^{-j(w_0 k+\theta_0)})) \tag{3}$$

where $\exp(x) \overset{def}{=} e^x$ and F(**z**) is a term independent of **u.**

The Cramer-Rao Lower Bound (CRLB) is the lowest value that can be attained by the variance of any unbiased estimator of **u** and is given by the diagonal elements of $\mathbf{J}_N^{-1}$ where

$\mathbf{J}_N$ is the Fisher information matrix defined by

$$\mathbf{J}_N = -E[\frac{\partial}{\partial \mathbf{u}}(\frac{\partial}{\partial \mathbf{u}} \ln(\mathrm{p}(\mathbf{z} \mid \mathbf{u})))^T] \tag{4}$$

Using (3), it can be shown that the error covariance matrix for joint frequency and phase estimation is lower-bounded by the 2x2 matrix

$$\mathbf{J}_N^{-1} = \frac{1/SNR}{N(N^2-1)} \begin{bmatrix} (N+1)(2N+1) & -3(N+1) \\ -3(N+1) & 6 \end{bmatrix} \tag{5}$$

where $SNR \overset{def}{=} \dfrac{1}{\sigma_v^{\ 2}}$ for BPSK. Therefore,

[1] For an M-PSK modulation, an *M*th order nonlinearity is required to remove the modulation [9].

$$CRLB_{\theta_0} = \mathbf{J}_N^{-1}(1,1) = \frac{(1/SNR)(2N+1)}{N(N-1)} \tag{6}$$

$$CRLB_{w_0} = \mathbf{J}_N^{-1}(2,2) = \frac{(6/SNR)}{N(N^2-1)} \tag{7}$$

It is interesting to note that the CRLB for random phase estimation decreases as $1/N$, while it decreases as $1/N^3$ for frequency estimation.

# 3. ALGORITHMS

While joint frequency and phase estimators have been developed [1,2], they are decision-directed (i.e. closed loop). Therefore, we restrict our discussion here to separate frequency and phase estimation algorithms.

## 3.1 Maximum Likelihood Frequency Estimation

The maximum likelihood estimate of $w_0$ is defined as follows

$$\hat{w}_{0,ML} = \arg\max_{w_0} p(\mathbf{z} \mid w_0) \tag{8}$$

It can be shown that $\hat{w}_{0,ML}$ is given by the frequency at which the periodogram of the noisy received signal attains its peak. Mathematically,

$$\hat{w}_{0,ML} = \arg\max_{w_0} \left| \sum_{k=1}^{N} z_k e^{-jw_0 k} \right|^2 \tag{9}$$

Although the computationally-efficient FFT algorithm can be used to compute the periodogram, accurate computation of $\hat{w}_{0,ML}$ still requires an exhaustive search and large storage requirements. Therefore, we investigate next several alternative Doppler frequency estimation algorithms that avoid this exhaustive search.

## 3.2 Tretter's Frequency Estimator

Equation (2) can be alternatively expressed as follows:

$$z_k = (1 + v_k e^{-j(w_0 k + \theta_0)}) e^{j(w_0 k + \theta_0)} \overset{def}{=} (1 + \eta_k) e^{j(w_0 k + \theta_0)} \tag{10}$$

where the complex-valued baseband noise samples $\eta_k = \Re(\eta_k) + j\Im(\eta_k)$ have variance $\sigma_\eta^2 = \sigma_v^2$. At high SNR (i.e. ${\sigma_\eta}^2 << 1$), we can write

$$1 + \eta_k \approx e^{j\Im(\eta_k)} \Rightarrow z_k \approx e^{j(w_0 k + \theta_0 + \Im(\eta_k))} \tag{11}$$

The above equation shows that at high SNR, the additive noise effects can be viewed as equivalent phase noise. Therefore, given the discrete samples $\mathbf{z}_k$, Tretter proposed in [8] to estimate $w_0$ and $\theta_0$ by performing a least-squares fit on the phase data

$$\phi_k = w_0 k + \theta_0 + \Im(\eta_k) \tag{12}$$

This, however, requires phase unwrapping that adds to the computational complexity and leads to high estimation errors due to cycle slips, especially at low signal-to-noise ratios.

## 3.3 Kay's Frequency Estimator

An elegant approach proposed in [6] avoids phase unwrapping by considering the *differenced* phase data. Using Equations (11) and (12)

$$\Delta_\Phi \overset{def}{=} \Phi_k - \Phi_{k-1} = \arg(z_k) - \arg(z_{k-1}) = \arg(z_k {z_{k-1}}^*) = w_0 + \Im(\eta_k) - \Im(\eta_{k-1}) \tag{13}$$

which describes a moving average process. It can be shown [6] that the maximum likelihood estimate of $w_0$ (which is also equivalent to the unbiased least squares estimate) is equal to

$$\hat{w}_0 = \frac{1}{2T} \sum_{k=1}^{N-1} g_k \arg(z_k z_{k-1}^*) \tag{14}$$

where the window $g_k$ is given by [6]

$$g_k = \frac{1.5N}{(N^2-1)}\left[1-\left(\frac{k-\left(N/2-1\right)}{N/2}\right)^2\right] \tag{15}$$

The variance of this frequency estimator, which we shall refer to as the *Kay estimator*, is given by

$$\mathrm{var}(\hat{w}_0) = \frac{6/SNR}{N(N^2-1)} \tag{16}$$

which achieves the Cramer-Rao bound (under the high-SNR assumption) and decreases as the cube of the packet length.

At high SNR, an equivalent frequency estimator can be derived by interchanging the argument and averaging operations, resulting in

$$\hat{w}_0 = \arg(\sum_{k=1}^{N-1} g_k z_k z_{k-1}^*) \tag{17}$$

At low to moderate SNR levels, the frequency estimator of (14) is superior to that of (17). It is also worth mentioning that for small frequency offsets $\left(w_0 << 1\right)$, the arg(.) function can be replaced by the $\Im(.)$ function to simplify the calculations. The Doppler frequency estimator of (17) will be referred to as the *high-SNR Kay estimator*

## 3.4 Fitz's Frequency Estimator

The time-varying nature of the window function in (15) makes a recursive high-speed implementation costly, especially for long packet lengths $N$. To reduce the cost while still retaining good performance, Fitz [3] proposed the use of higher-order lags for the sample auto-correlation function of $\mathbf{z}_k$. The rationale behind this is as follows. The argument of the signal component in the $m^{th}$ order lag is linearly proportional to $m$ while the noise has the same statistical description for all lags. This results in a more accurate frequency estimator. Mathematically, the Doppler frequency estimator can be derived by taking the derivative of the periodogram function (given by the right hand side of Equation (9)) with respect to $w_0$ and setting the result to zero. This results in the optimality condition

$$\Im\left(\sum_{m=1}^{N} mR_z(m)e^{-jw_0 m}\right) = 0 \tag{18}$$

Next, we make the following (high SNR) assumption

$$\Im(R_z(m)e^{-jw_0 k}) \approx \arg(R_z(m)) - w_0 k \tag{19}$$

This assumption allows us to approximate the likelihood equation of (18) as follows

$$\sum_{m=1}^{N} m(\arg(R_z(m)) - mw_0 k) \approx 0 \tag{20}$$

Truncating the sum at the $J^{\text{th}}$ term, Fitz proposed the following frequency estimator [3]

$$\hat{w}_0 = \frac{\sum_{m=1}^{J} m \arg(R_z(m))}{\sum_{m=1}^{J} m^2}$$

$$= \frac{6}{J(J+1)(2J+1)} \sum_{m=1}^{J} m \arg(R_z(m))$$

$$= \sum_{m=1}^{J} C(J,m) \arg(R_z(m)) \tag{21}$$

where $R_z(m) = \sum_{k=m+1}^{N} z_k z_{k-m}^*$ is the sample auto-correlation sequence and $J$ is typically $\leq 3$. This Doppler frequency estimator will be referred to as the *Fitz estimator*. We conclude this section by mentioning that uniformly-spaced samples have been assumed throughout. Doppler frequency estimation with non-uniformly spaced samples is treated in [4].

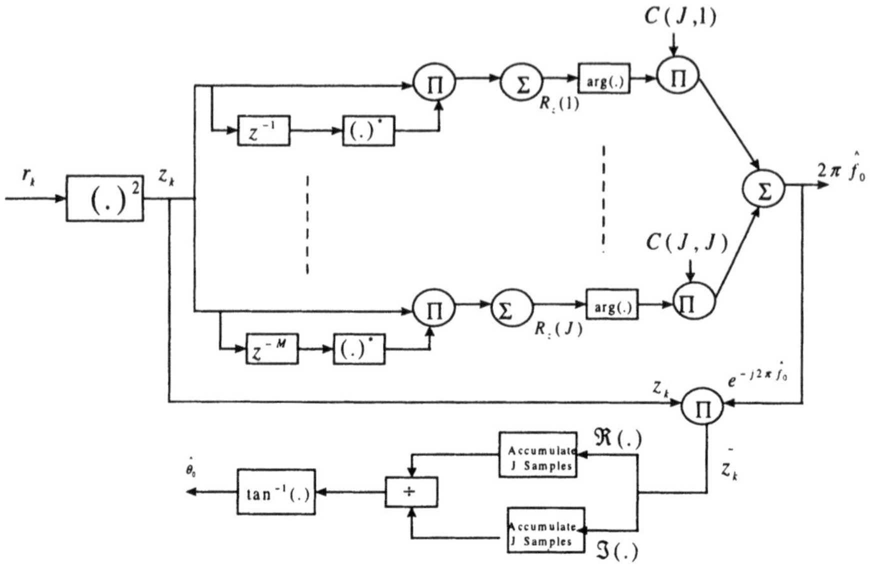


*Figure 21.* Frequency and Phase Estimators of Fitz.

## 3.5 Random Phase Estimation

The next step is to estimate the random phase offset $\theta_0$ which is assumed to be constant over the packet. The methods of the previous section are used to remove the frequency error resulting in the discrete-time samples

$$\begin{aligned} \tilde{z}_k &= z_k e^{-j\hat{w}_0 k} \\ &= e^{jk(w_0-\hat{w}_0)} e^{j\theta_0} + \tilde{v}_k \end{aligned} \tag{22}$$

Assuming accurate frequency offset estimation, i.e., $\hat{w}_0 \approx w_0$, then

$$\tilde{z}_k \approx e^{j\theta_0} + \tilde{v}_k \tag{23}$$

The ML estimate of $\theta_0$ is given by

$$\hat{\theta}_0 = \arg\max_{\theta_0} p(\tilde{\mathbf{z}} \mid \theta_0) \tag{24}$$

where

$$p(\tilde{\mathbf{z}} \mid \theta_0) = F(\tilde{\mathbf{z}}) \exp\left( \frac{2}{\sigma_v^2} \sum_{k=1}^{N} \Re(\tilde{z}_k e^{-j\theta_0}) \right)$$

is the conditional pdf of $\tilde{\mathbf{z}} \overset{def}{=} [\tilde{z}_0, \tilde{z}_1, \cdots, \tilde{z}_{N-1}]$ given $\theta_0$. Setting $\frac{\partial p(\tilde{\mathbf{z}} \mid \theta_0)}{\partial \theta_0} = 0$, we get

$$\sum_{k=1}^{N} \Im(\tilde{z}_k e^{-j\theta_0}) = 0 \Rightarrow (\sum_{k=1}^{N} \Im(\tilde{z}_k)) \cos(\theta_0) = (\sum_{k=1}^{N} \Re(\tilde{z}_k)) \sin(\theta_0) \quad (25)$$

which leads to the following simple technique for estimating $\theta_0$

$$\hat{\theta}_0 = \tan^{-1} \left( \frac{\sum_{k=1}^{J} \Im(\tilde{z}_k)}{\sum_{k=1}^{J} \Re(\tilde{z}_k)} \right) \quad (26)$$

*Figure 21* depicts the frequency and phase estimators of Equation (21) and (26), respectively.

# 4. SIMULATION RESULTS

In this section, we evaluate the performance of three Doppler frequency estimators described in the previous section; namely the Kay estimator, the high-SNR Kay estimator, and the Fitz estimator. The performance metric adopted is the Root-Mean-Square (RMS) Doppler frequency error defined as follows

$$w_{0,error}^{RMS} = \sqrt{\frac{1}{N_b} \sum_{i=1}^{N_b} (\hat{w}_{0,i} - w_{0,i})^2} \quad (27)$$

where $w_{0,i}$ is the Doppler frequency offset of the $i$-th burst, $\hat{w}_{0,i}$ is its estimate, and $N_b$ is the number of received data bursts.

As a performance benchmark, we also compute the Cramer-Rao lower bound on frequency estimation given by

$$CRLB_{w_0} = \frac{6/SNR}{N(N^2-1)} \tag{28}$$

In our computer simulations, we assume BPSK packet transmission on an AWGN channel with constant normalized Doppler frequency offset $w_0 = 0.5$ and random phase error $\theta \in [0^0, 360^0]$ assumed constant throughout each packet.

The three frequency estimators are computed on a packet-by-packet basis, and the RMS statistic in (24) is calculated by averaging over 1000 bursts.

*Figure 22* through *Figure 24* depict the variation of the estimated Doppler frequency over the 1000 received bursts for the Kay, high-SNR Kay, and Fitz estimators, respectively. We assume a packet length $N$ = 128 bits and operating SNR = 15 dB.

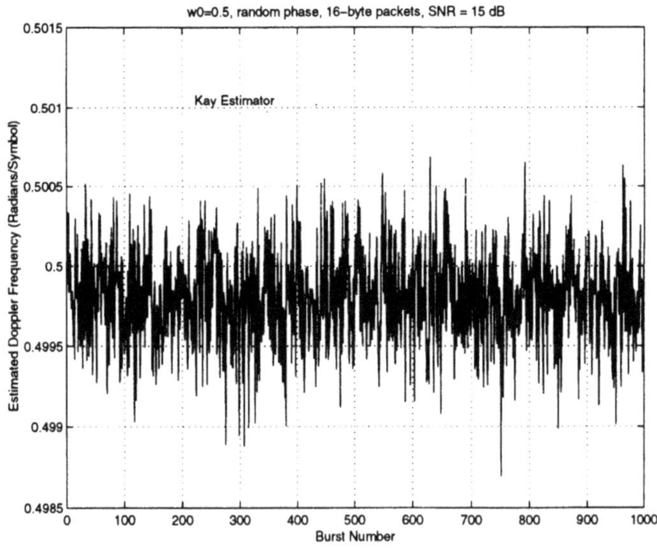


*Figure 22*. Estimated Doppler Frequency using Kay's Estimator for 1000 bursts

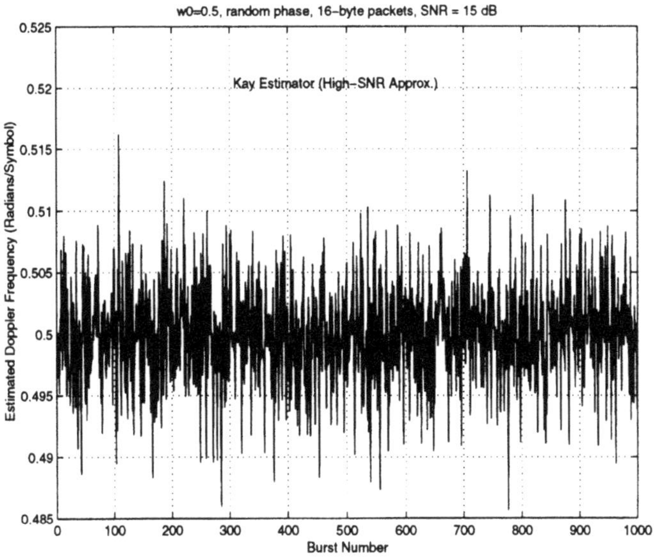


*Figure 23.* Estimated Doppler Frequency using High-SNR Kay's Estimator for 1000 bursts.

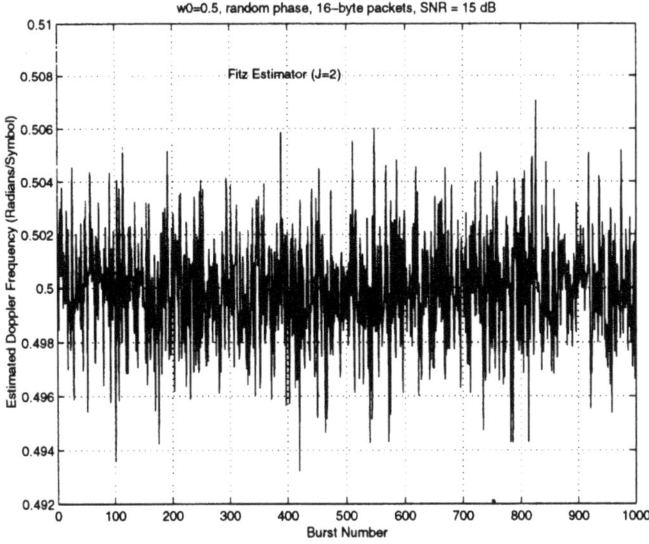


*Figure 24.* Estimated Doppler Frequency using Fitz Estimator for 1000 bursts.

The variation of the RMS Doppler frequency error (in degrees) versus SNR for the three frequency estimators is shown in *Figure 25* and compared with the Cramer-Rao lower bound. The assumed packet length is 128 bits. It can be seen that all three estimators converge to the Cramer-Rao bound at high SNR. At low SNR, their performance deteriorates rapidly, due to the well-known threshold effect experienced by non-linear single-frequency estimators [7].

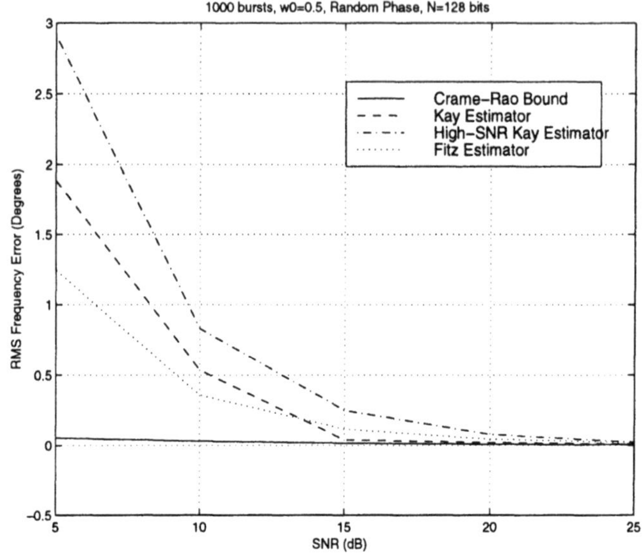


*Figure 25.* RMS Frequency Error (in degrees) versus SNR for the Three Frequency Estimators and the Cramer-Rao Lower Bound.

We conclude this section by mentioning that the RMS Doppler frequency error also decreases with increasing packet length, since more observations are used to compute the estimator. This effect is shown in *Figure 26*.

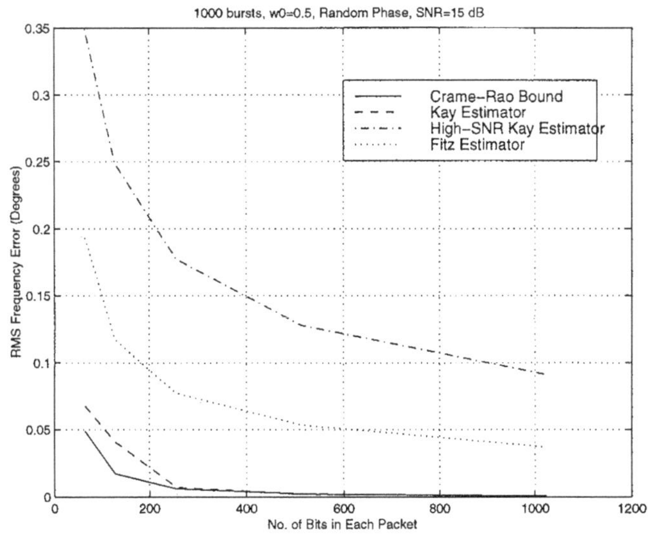


*Figure 26.* RMS Frequency Error (in degrees) versus Packet Length for the Three Frequency Estimators and the Cramer-Rao Lower Bound.

# REFERENCES


[1] M. Fitz, "Planar Filtered Techniques for Burst Mode Carrier Synchronization," *Proc. GLOBECOM'91*, p. 12.1.1-12.1.5

[2] M. Fitz and W. Lindsey, "Decision-Directed Burst-Mode Carrier Synchronization Techniques," *IEEE Transactions on Communications*, October 1992, p. 1644-1653.

[3] M. Fitz, "Further Results in the Fast Estimation of a Single Frequency," *IEEE Transactions on Communications*, Feb/March/April 1994, p. 862-864.

[4] J. Gansman, K. Krogmeier, M. Fitz, and A. Singh, "Single Frequency Estimation with Non-Uniform Sampling," *Proceedings of the Asilomar Conference on Signals, Systems, and Computers*, November 1996, p. 399-403.

[5] F. Gardner, "Hangup in Phase-Lock Loops," *IEEE Transactions on Communications*, October 1977, p. 1210-1214.

[6] S. Kay, "A Fast and Accurate Single Frequency Estimator," *IEEE Transactions on Acoustics, Speech, and Signal Processing*, December 1989, p. 1987-1990.

[7] D. Rife, "Single-Tone Parameter Estimation from Discrete-Time Observations," *IEEE Transactions on Information Theory*, September 1974, p. 591-598.

[8] S. Tretter, "Estimating the Frequency of a Noisy Sinusoid by Linear Regression," *IEEE Transactions on Information Theory*, December 1985, p. 832-835.

[9] A. Viterbi and A. Viterbi, "Nonlinear Estimation of PSK-Modulated Carrier Phase with Application to Burst Digital Transmission," *IEEE Transactions on Information Theory*, July 1983, p. 543-551.

# Chapter 4

# Satellite Visibility Prediction

In this chapter, we present a simple algorithm to determine the visibility-time function at a given location on Earth for circular LEO satellites. Numerical results show that for a wide range of LEO orbit altitudes, the algorithm provides accurate results for predicting the satellite's rise time and in-view period. The algorithm implemented in the mobile terminal's processor could be used to aid power conservation and communication functions in the mobile.

## 1. INTRODUCTION

A variety of LEO satellite systems have recently been proposed for personal communications [1]. In these systems, satellites follow inclined circular orbits with altitudes between 600 km and 1400 km. These systems provide global communications capability; however, at any given location on Earth, a LEO satellite is visible only for a short duration of time. For example, the length of the maximum in-view period is under 15 minutes for a satellite at 1000 km altitude.

Predicting the visibility of LEO satellites at a terminal is valuable for a number of reasons. By implementing the visibility prediction algorithm at a terminal, the terminal could conserve power by going into a power conserving "sleep" mode until the next rise time of the satellite. Also, for communication through LEO satellites, it is beneficial for the terminal to communicate with the satellite when the elevation angle to the satellite is large. This is because there is lower probability of line-of-sight blockage, and the slant range to the satellite is shorter, providing a better communication channel. The in-view period varies between satellite passes and is a function of the maximum elevation angle between the terminal and the satellite during a satellite pass; the greater the maximum elevation angle to the satellite, the longer the in-view period. Thus the terminal could improve the probability of successful communication with a satellite by transmitting during the middle of a longer in-view period pass of the satellite.

The visibility prediction algorithm presented in this chapter uses a result we derived in Chapter 2 for circular orbit LEO satellites that relates the maximum observed elevation angle during a satellite pass to the length of the in-view period. The maximum elevation angle is observed at the instant the sub-satellite point is closest to the terminal. To compute the location of this point and the epoch of its occurrence without resorting to exhaustive orbit propagation, we approximate the ground trace of the satellite during the in-view period by a great-circle arc. In reality, the ground trace of a LEO satellite deviates from a great-circle arc due to Earth's rotation. However, in [5] we showed that using the great-circle arc approximation at LEO altitudes provided very accurate results for the Doppler time curve observed at a terminal. Here we use the great-circle arc approximation to enable the use of spherical geometry to efficiently compute the sub-satellite point closest to the terminal and the corresponding epoch of its occurrence. The algorithm provides accurate results even for LEO satellite orbits at relatively high altitudes.

In the literature, two approaches for computing the visibility-time function of satellites have been reported in [2,3]. In [2], the authors apply orbit propagation routines on the satellite constellation to obtain the visibility-time function. Orbit propagation is the predominant method of determining satellite visibility. Visibility prediction through orbit propagation involves mathematically generating the satellite's orbit, sampled on a fine time grid. Visibility conditions are determined for each time sample. This process is computationally intensive. The visibility prediction algorithm that we introduce here avoids exhaustive enumeration by using approximations to determine the satellite visibility data. In [3], the satellite visibility prediction algorithm is a small but integral part of a design methodology for LEO satellite systems. The authors use an iterative approach, similar to the one used here, to determine in-view period. For each rotation of the satellite, the algorithm solves an analytic expression to determine whether the satellite is visible at the terminal or not. If the satellite visibility condition is met, the algorithm determines the in-view period by computing the satellite's rise and set time at the terminal. The algorithm used in [3] uses expressions that are valid in the ECI reference frame but assumes that the terminal is fixed and not moving as the Earth rotates. To correct for this assumption, successive approximations, which update the terminal's location at computed rise and set times, are used. By contrast, the algorithm presented here explicitly accounts for the movement of the terminal due to Earth's rotation.

# 2. VISIBILITY PREDICTION ALGORITHM

## 2.1 Algorithm Overview

We provide an overview of the algorithm with the help of *Figure 27*. *Figure 27* shows one visibility pass of an Orbcomm satellite (altitude = 738 km, inclination = $70^0$, and eccentricity assumed to be zero) at a terminal, located at $39^0N$ latitude and $77^0W$ longitude. For a satellite to be visible to the terminal, the ground trace of the satellite should be within the visibility perimeter. The minimum elevation angle required for visibility, denoted $\theta_c$, is assumed to be $10^0$ in the figure.

The visibility-time profile is computed by iterating over consecutive rotations of the satellite. For each satellite rotation, the algorithm determines whether the satellite is visible to the terminal; if so, it computes an accurate approximation for the maximum elevation angle from the terminal to the satellite and the time instant of observation of the maximum elevation angle.

Determining if a satellite is visible to a terminal in a particular rotation of the satellite is complicated by the fact that the terminal moves due to the Earth's rotation. In a frame of reference fixed to the Earth, the ECF frame, the terminal is stationary, but the path of the satellite is not a great circle and hence spherical geometry relations cannot be used. However, if one approximates a small segment of the ground trace of a LEO satellite by a great-circle arc, simple analytic expressions can be used to determine the visibility condition and the in-view period. In [5], we showed that the error in approximating a segment of the ground trace of a LEO satellite over a period equal to the maximum visibility of the satellite at a terminal is very small. However, since the great-circle arc approximation is only valid for short ground trace segments, to determine in-view period we should approximate the satellite's ground trace when it is in close vicinity of the terminal. For inclined orbit satellites, an easy way to compute coordinates on the ground trace of a satellite in close proximity to the terminal's location is by first determining the intersection of the ground trace with the terminal's latitude. By computing two points close to this intersection, we obtain the expression for the great-circle arc approximation. These points are represented by the two 'x's in *Figure 27*. Using a simple geometric relation we compute the point on the great-circle arc approximation that is closest to the terminal, i.e., a point on the great-circle arc from which the distance to the terminal is the shortest. A corresponding point on the ground trace is computed. This point is shown by the 'o' in *Figure 27*. At this point on the ground trace the central angle between the sub-satellite point and the terminal is at its minimum value. If the satellite is visible to the terminal, the central angle should be within a specified range, i.e., the point of closest approach should be within the visibility perimeter shown in *Figure 27*. Also, at this point of closest approach, the elevation angle from the terminal to the satellite is at its maximum value and can be easily computed (Equation (13)). Using results from [5], we determine the in-view period from the maximum elevation angle, and since the visibility window is centered at the epoch of observation of the maximum elevation angle, we are able to determine the rising and setting epochs of the satellite.

The inputs to the algorithm are orbit parameters describing the satellite path, and also an initial reference location of the satellite. The results of the algorithm are with respect to these initial space-time coordinates. Time within each iteration of the algorithm is measured with respect to some conveniently chosen space-time instant representing the beginning of an iteration. The space-time instant we choose to represent the beginning of a cycle is the instant at which the satellite's ground trace crosses the equator with the satellite transitioning from the southern hemisphere to the northern hemisphere.

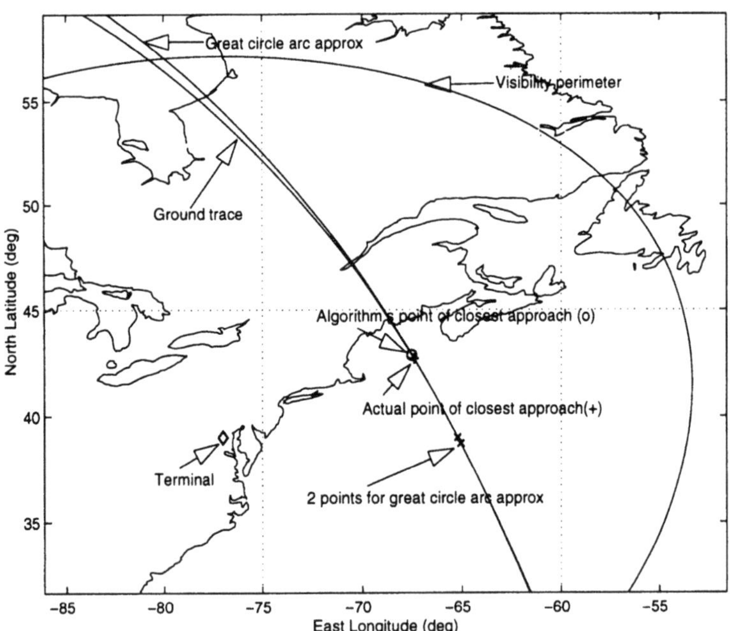


*Figure 27*. An illustration of the mechanics of the algorithm for one satellite pass. Satellite orbit's altitude is 738 km and inclination $69^0$.

## 2.2 Detailed Algorithm

### 2.2.1 Inputs

The inputs to our algorithm are:

1. *Orbital parameters*: Orbit radius ($r$) or orbit period ($T_s$) or ECI angular velocity ($\omega_s$) and orbit inclination ($i$).
2. *Initial location of the satellite*: Time instant ($t_0$) and longitude ($\lambda_0$), of the satellite in the equatorial plane when transitioning from the southern hemisphere to the northern hemisphere.
3. *Location of the terminal*: Longitude($\lambda_t$) and latitude ($\phi_t$) of the terminal's location. Vector $\mathbf{x}_t$ denotes the coordinates of the terminal in the Cartesian frame.

The specific input values for most commercial LEO satellites can be obtained from NASA's Web site [6]. Using calculations [4, pg. 127-130], one can obtain the satellite's terrestrial latitude, $\phi_0$, and longitude, $\lambda_0$, at the given time epoch $t_0^{'}$ specified in the database. However, the input to our algorithm requires that at the initial time epoch the satellite be at the equator, i.e., $\phi_0 = 0$. The generalization to cover the case when the initial latitude location of the satellite is arbitrary leads to a more complex expression in Step 1 of our algorithm, detailed below. Since Step 1 is repeated for each rotation of the satellite, it is simpler to restrict the initial latitude of the satellite to the equator and compute the corresponding time epoch, $t_0$, for this location. To do this, we first compute the time $\Delta t_0$ it took the satellite to propagate from the equator to its current phase in the circular orbit given by $(\alpha + M_0)$, where $\alpha$ is the argument of perigee and $M_0$ is the mean anomaly at the time epoch. These parameters are provided by the NASA database. Assuming a circular orbit satellite, $\Delta t_0 = (\alpha + M_0)^{T_s}/_{2\pi}$. The corresponding initial time epoch input to the algorithm is $t_0 = t_0^{'} - \Delta t_0$. The longitude of the sub-satellite point at the equator can be obtained from the right ascension of the ascending node ($\Omega$) parameter provided in the database by

$$\lambda_0 = \Omega - \mathrm{GMST}(t_0) \tag{1}$$

where GMST($t_0$) is the Greenwich mean sidereal time at $t_0$.

### 2.2.2 Outputs

The outputs are in the form of two sequences:

1. Sequence of maximum elevation angles $\{\theta_1, \theta_2, \theta_3, \ldots, \theta_n\}$.
2. Sequence of maximum elevation angle observation instants $\{u_1, u_2, \ldots, u_n\}$.

In [5], we derived an accurate analytic approximation for the satellite in-view period, $\tau(\theta_{\max})$, as a function of the maximum elevation angle,

$$\tau(\theta_{\max}) \approx \frac{2}{\omega_s - \omega_E \cos i} \cos^{-1}\left( \frac{\cos\left(\cos^{-1}\left(\frac{r_E}{r}\cos\theta_c\right) - \theta_c\right)}{\cos\left(\cos^{-1}\left(\frac{r_E}{r}\cos\theta_{\max}\right) - \theta_{\max}\right)} \right) \tag{2}$$

where the parameters are

- $\theta_{\max}$ maximum elevation angle during the visibility window,
- $\theta_c$ minimum elevation angle for visibility,
- $r_E$ radius of the Earth,
- $r$ radius of the satellite's orbit,
- $\omega_s$ angular velocity of the satellite in the ECI frame,
- $\omega_E$ angular velocity of the Earth's rotation,
- $i$ inclination of the satellite's orbit.

Thus the satellite in-view periods are $\tau(\theta_k)$, $k = 1, \ldots, n$. The visibility window is centered at the maximum elevation angle observation instant. Hence, the visibility time function for the satellite is

$$v(t) = \begin{cases} 1 & \text{if } t \in \left[u_k - \frac{\tau(\theta_k)}{2}, u_k + \frac{\tau(\theta_k)}{2}\right], \quad k = 1, \ldots, n \\ 0 & \text{otherwise} \end{cases} \tag{3}$$

### 2.2.3 Steps of the Algorithm

The following variables are used by the algorithm:

- $T_{i,0}$ time instant at the start of the $i$-th rotation,
- $\lambda_{i,0}$ longitude of the intersection of the satellite's orbit with the equatorial plane at the start of the $i$-th rotation,
- $t$ time within a rotation. $t = 0$ at the start of a rotation.

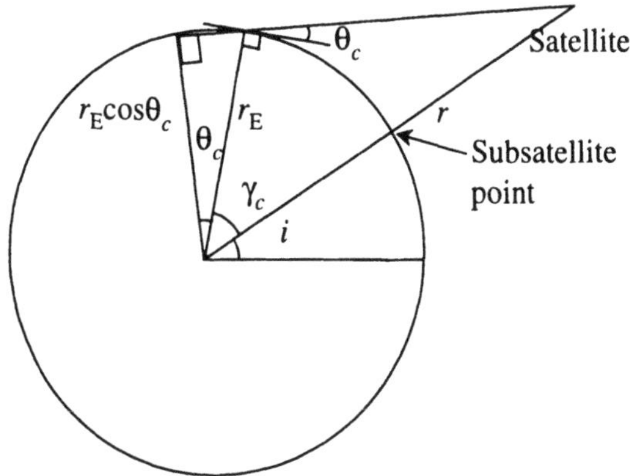


*Figure 28.* Determination of the coverage region for a circular orbit LEO satellite.

1. *Determine if the terminal is within the satellite's coverage latitudes*: Inclined orbit LEO satellites are visible from within a latitude range on the Earth's surface. The latitude range depends on the inclination of the orbit, the altitude of the orbit, and the minimum elevation angle required for visibility. The coverage region, expressed in terms of latitude degrees, is given by [max(-90,$-i-\gamma_c$), min(90, $i+\gamma_c$)], where $\gamma_c$ is the central angle between a point on the Earth at the edge of satellite's visibility and the sub-satellite point. From *Figure 28*, $\gamma_c$ is given by

$$\gamma_c = \cos^{-1}\left(\frac{r_E}{r}\cos\theta_c\right) - \theta_c \tag{4}$$

If the terminal is not located in the coverage region, the satellite will never be visible to the terminal, and we quit the algorithm.

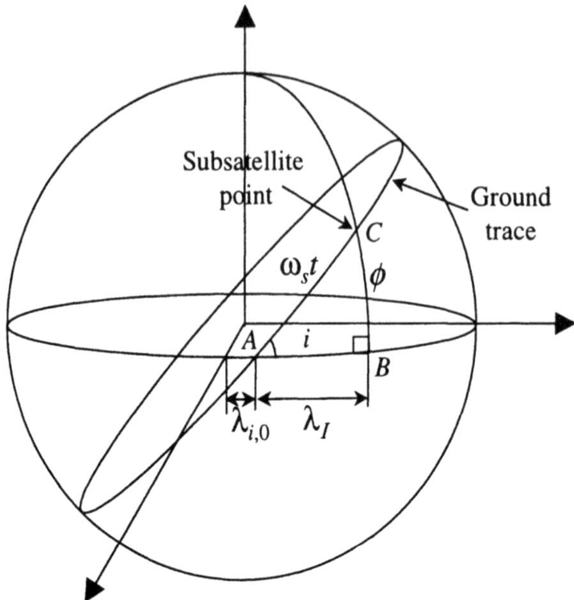


*Figure 29.* Geometrical relation between the sub-satellite point's latitude and longitude in the ECI coordinate frame.

For rotation $i$=1,2,3,...

2. *Determine the intersection of the satellite's orbit with the terminal's latitude*: If the terminal is located within the coverage region but not within the range [$-i$,$i$] latitude, the ground trace of the satellite does not intersect the terminal's latitude. In this case we compute the intersection of the ground trace with either $+i$ or $-i$ degrees latitude depending on whether the terminal is located in the northern hemisphere or the southern hemisphere, respectively.
   From spherical trigonometry, using sine and cosine laws to the spherical triangle *ABC* in *Figure 29*, the equations relating the sub-satellite point's latitude, $\phi$, and longitude ($\lambda_I + \lambda_{i,0}$) in the ECI coordinate system are given by

$$\sin\phi(t) = \sin i \sin\omega_s t \tag{5}$$

$$\cos\omega_s t = \cos\lambda_I(t)\cos\phi(t) \tag{6}$$

To compute the sub-satellite point's longitude in the ECF frame, $\lambda$, we compensate for the Earth's rotation to give

$$\lambda(t) = \lambda_I(t) + \lambda_{i,0} - \omega_E t \tag{7}$$

The time instant, $t_a$, and the longitude, $\lambda_a$, of the intersection of the ground trace with the terminal's latitude is obtained from,

$$\omega_s t_a = \eta \stackrel{\Delta}{=} \sin^{-1}\left(\frac{\sin\phi_t}{\sin i}\right) \tag{8}$$

$$\lambda_a = \cos^{-1}\left(\frac{\cos\omega_s t_a}{\cos\phi_t}\right) - \omega_E t_a + \lambda_{i,0} \tag{9}$$

The right hand side of Equation (8) has two solutions, as the ground trace intersects the terminal's latitude at two points. In one case the satellite is approaching the equator and in the other case the satellite is receding from the equator. Assuming that the $\sin^{-1}(\theta)$ function returns values in the range $[-\pi/2,+\pi/2]$, the two solutions for Equation (8) are $pv(\eta,\pi-\eta)$ where $pv(\theta)$ is a function that returns the principal value of an angle in the range $[0,2\pi]$. From the two solutions, we choose that intersection of the ground trace which is closer to the terminal's longitude.

3. *Compute the great-circle arc approximation of the ground trace and the minimum perpendicular distance to the terminal*: Two points on the ground trace at times $t_a$ and $t_b = t_a + \Delta t$ are used to define the great-circle arc. Using Equation (5) through (7), we compute the sub-satellite points, denoted by vectors $\mathbf{x}_a$ and $\mathbf{x}_b$, at these two time instances. The unit vector perpendicular to the plane defined by ($\mathbf{x}_a$, $\mathbf{x}_b$, 0), denoted by $\mathbf{n}$, is

$$\mathbf{n} = \frac{\mathbf{x}_a \times \mathbf{x}_b}{|\mathbf{x}_a \times \mathbf{x}_b|} \tag{10}$$

The perpendicular distance of the terminal from the plane defined by the great-circle arc approximation is $p = \mathbf{x}_t \cdot \mathbf{n}$ and the central angle between the terminal and the point on the great-circle arc approximation closest to the terminal is given by

$$\gamma = \sin^{-1}\left(\frac{p}{r_E}\right) \tag{11}$$

4. *Compute time instant of closest approach*: The location of the sub-satellite point at the instant of maximum elevation angle observation, denoted by $\hat{\mathbf{x}}_{\mathbf{m}}$ is

$$\hat{\mathbf{x}}_{\mathbf{m}} = \frac{1}{\cos\gamma}(\mathbf{x}_{\mathbf{t}} - p\mathbf{n}) \tag{12}$$

Let $(\hat{\lambda}_m, \hat{\phi}_m)$ denote the longitude and latitude corresponding to the location $\hat{\mathbf{x}}_{\mathbf{m}}$. Note that $(\hat{\lambda}_m, \hat{\phi}_m)$ is an approximation of the sub-satellite point at the instant of maximum elevation angle observation based on the great-circle arc approximation of the ground trace. This point might not lie on the actual ground trace, i.e., $(\hat{\lambda}_m, \hat{\phi}_m)$ might not satisfy Equations (5), (6), and (7) simultaneously. We compute the time $t_m$ when the sub-satellite point is at latitude $\hat{\phi}_m$ from Equation (5). Note that $\hat{\phi}_m$ should be constrained to lie in the range $[-i,i]$ latitude.

5. *Refine the estimates*: To refine the estimates of the time instant of maximum elevation angle observation, we approximate the ground trace closer to the point of closest approach. For this, we use two points on the ground trace at times $t_m$ and $t_m + \Delta t$ to define the great-circle arc. Steps 2 and 3 are repeated to provide more accurate estimates of $\gamma$ and $t_m$. Note that this step is not illustrated in *Figure 27*, but is very important in improving the algorithm's accuracy when the point of closest approach on the ground trace is much further away from the intersection of the ground trace with the terminal's latitude. An example of such a case is shown in *Figure 30*. There one can observe that the first great-circle arc approximation deviates significantly from the ground trace at the point of closest approach. The second great-circle arc approximation is much closer to the ground trace at the point of closest approach.

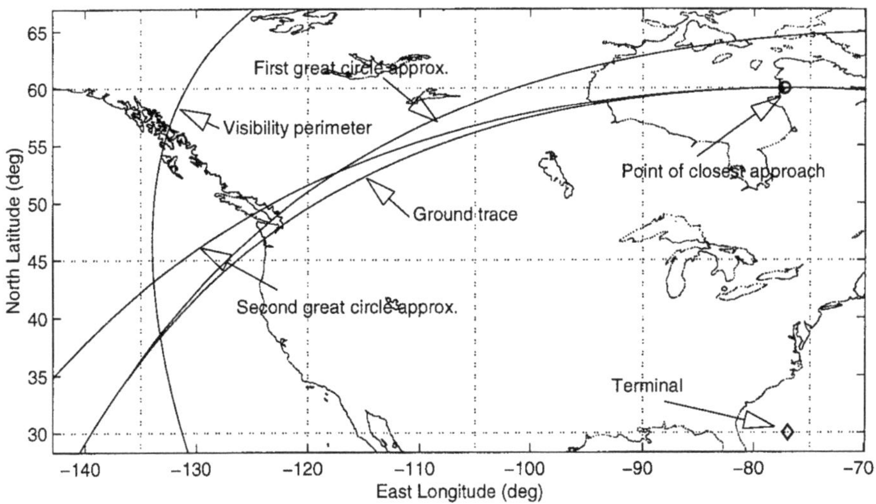


*Figure 30.* Illustration of the scenario when the point of closest approach on the ground trace is far from the intersection of the ground trace with the terminal's latitude. Satellite's orbit altitude is 5000 km and the inclination is $60^0$.

6. *Check satellite visibility condition*: If the satellite is visible to the terminal, the elevation angle from the terminal to the satellite should be greater than the minimum elevation angle for visibility, $\theta_c$. The condition on $\gamma$ for visibility is $-\gamma_c \leq \gamma \leq \gamma_c$, where $\gamma_c$ is given by Equation (4). If this condition is not met, the satellite is not visible during the current rotation, and we go to Step 8 of the algorithm.
7. *Compute the maximum elevation angle*: At the point of closest approach of the ground trace to the terminal, the central angle between the terminal and the ground trace is minimum. At this instant, the elevation angle from the terminal to the satellite is maximum. The maximum elevation angle, $\theta_{max}$, is given by [4, Equation (3-4)]

$$\theta_{max} = \cos^{-1}\left(\frac{r_E \sin\gamma}{\sqrt{r_E^2 + r^2 - 2r_E r\cos\gamma}}\right) \tag{13}$$

8. *Save results and update variables for next rotation*: If the satellite is visible during the current rotation, the actual time for the observation of the maximum elevation angle of the satellite is

$$u_k = T_{i,0} + t_m \tag{14}$$

and $\theta_k = \theta_{max}$. For the next rotation of the satellite

$$T_{i+1,0} = T_{i,0} + T_s \tag{15}$$

The longitude of the intersection of the ground trace with the equator for the ($i$+1)-th rotation is

$$\lambda_{i+1,0} = \lambda_{i,0} - \omega_E T_s \tag{16}$$

Go to Step 2 to compute results for ($i$+1)-th rotation of the satellite.

## 3. NUMERICAL RESULTS

We consider circular LEO satellite orbits at altitudes of 1000 km and 5000 km above the Earth's surface, and orbit inclination $60^0$. The location on the Earth's surface at which we compute the visibility-time function is $30^0$ *N* and $77^0$ *W*. The minimum elevation angle for visibility is $10^0$. An orbit generation program written in MATLAB® was used to obtain the exact results. The program generates satellite orbits, sampled 16,000 times each day (5.4 sec sampling interval), for a duration of 10 days. Higher order perturbation effects are ignored, under the assumption that satellite stationkeeping will result in circular orbits.

In *Figure 31*, we plot the percentage normalized error in predicting the satellite rise time. This error is defined as

$$\%\ \text{Normlized Error} = \frac{(\text{Predicted satellite rise time} - \text{Actual satellite rise time})}{\text{Actual in - view period}} \times 100 \tag{17}$$

Defined in this manner, the normalized error gives the error in predicting the satellite rise time as a percentage of the satellite visibility time during the particular satellite pass. The in-view period is a function of the maximum elevation angle observable during a satellite pass. Thus, for lower maximum elevation angle, the same error in predicting satellite rise time leads to higher normalized error value. The percentage normalized error is plotted as a function of the maximum elevation angle observed during the visibility window. The data cover the entire range of maximum elevation angles from $10^0$ to $90^0$.

® MATLAB is a registered trademark of The MathWorks, Inc.

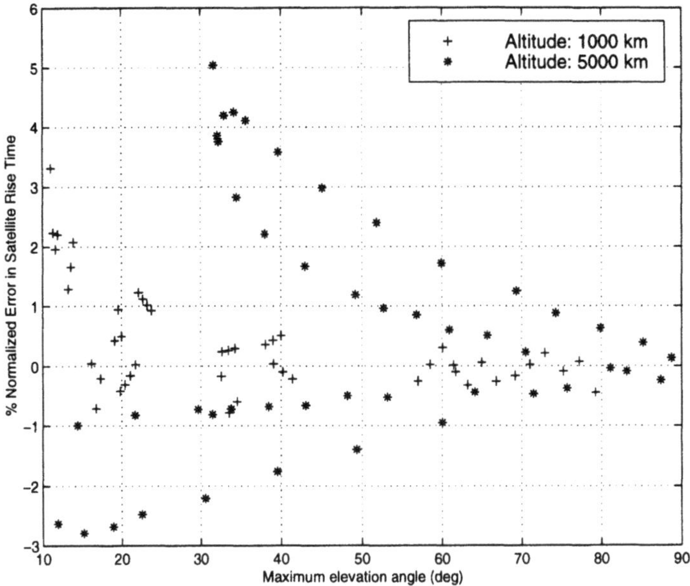


*Figure 31.* Percentage normalized error in predicting the satellite's rise time as a function of the maximum elevation angle observable during the satellite's pass for orbit altitudes 1000 km and 5000 km and inclination $60^0$.

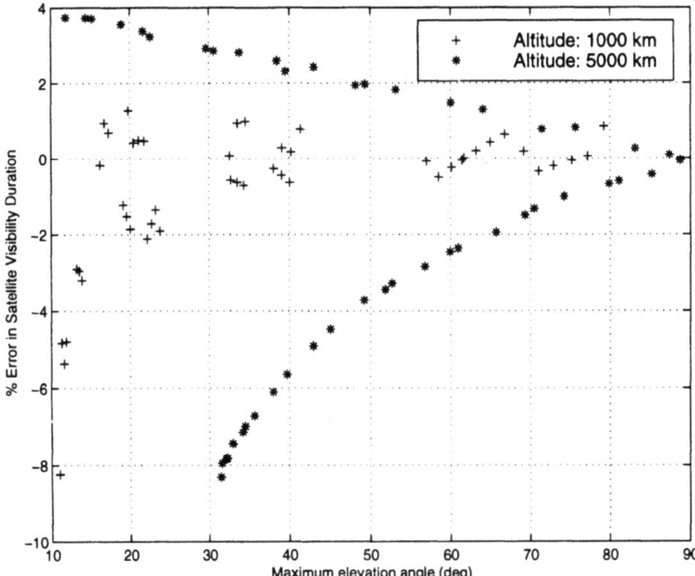


*Figure 32.* Percentage error in predicting in-view period as a function of the maximum elevation angle observable during the satellite's pass for orbit altitudes 1000 km and 5000 km and inclination $60^0$.

In *Figure 32*, we plot the percentage error in the algorithm for predicting the in-view period as a function of the maximum elevation angle. The percentage error in both these figures decreases with maximum elevation angle as the in-view period, which is the normalizing factor in both the error computations, increases with the maximum elevation angle.

The percentage error in the prediction of the in-view period increases with the orbit's altitude. With an increase in the orbit altitude, the period of rotation of the satellite increases. This causes a greater deviation of the ground trace from a great-circle arc due to the increased effect of Earth's rotation. Also, with an increase in the orbit's altitude, for the same maximum elevation angle, the in-view period of satellite increases (in Equation (1), the denominator $\omega_s$ decreases with altitude). For these two reasons, the satellite's ground trace during the in-view period deviates to a greater extent from a great-circle arc approximation for higher satellite altitudes. The deviation, in turn, increases the error in the overall algorithm's results.

A caveat to note is that very infrequently, at certain terminal locations, the algorithm fails to predict a satellite's pass with very short in-view period. The maximum elevation angles for these passes are within $3^0$ of the cutoff visibility elevation angle. This happens in those cases when the ground trace of the satellite grazes the terminal's visibility perimeter at a latitude far from the terminal's latitude. However, low visibility passes that occur in close vicinity of the terminal's latitude are accurately predicted by the algorithm.

## REFERENCES

[1] B. Miller, "Satellites Free the Mobile Phone," *IEEE Spectrum*, Vol. 35, No. 3, March 1998, p. 26-35.

[2] T. J. Lang and J. M. Hanson, "Orbital Constellations which Minimize Revisit Time," *AAS*, vol. 83-402, p. 1071-1086.

[3] J. Radzik and G. Maral, "A Methodology for Rapidly Evaluating the Performance of Some Low Earth Orbit Satellite Systems," *IEEE Journal on Selected Areas in Communications*, Vol. 13, No. 2, February 19956, p. 301-309.

[4] W.L. Pritchard, H.G. Suyderhoud and R.A. Nelson, *Satellite Communication Systems Engineering*, Prentice Hall, 1993.

[5] I. Ali, N. Al-Dhahir, and J. E. Hershey, "Doppler Characterization for LEO Satellites," *IEEE Transactions on Communications*, Vol. 46, No. 3, March 1998, p. 309-313.

[6] http://oig1.gsfc.nasa.gov. NASA's web site for orbit parameters of satellites.

# Chapter 5

# Doppler Based Multiple Access

In this chapter, we show how to use the Doppler-time S-curve, observed by terminals on the outbound downlink channel (from satellite to terminal) due to the relative motion between the satellite and the terminal, in a novel way to provide flow control in a LEO satellite messaging communication system. The control scheme, Doppler Based Multiple Access, or DBMA, uses two parameters of the Doppler S-curve, namely, maximum elevation angle and zero-Doppler time, to specify a region of eligibility (ROE) for transmission from terminals. Only terminals inside the ROE are allowed to transmit. The size of the ROE can be modified by controlling two parameters to provide a highly effective flow control method for traffic on the inbound channel. Through computer simulations, we illustrate the effectiveness of DBMA. We also show that quadratic curve fitting of Doppler frequency measurements is fairly accurate for a wide range of maximum elevation angles. DBMA promises to be a powerful and effective method for flow control for LEO satellite systems.

## 1. INTRODUCTION

This chapter is concerned only with a subclass of LEO satellites. This subclass is termed the "Little" LEOs. They are typically LEO satellites that provide a narrow class of low bandwidth aperiodic services such as messaging. Further, this Little LEO subclass can be partitioned into those Little LEO satellites that accomplish their mission with onboard memory in what is termed "store-and-forward" operation; and those Little LEOs that function as a "bent pipe," i.e., have an onboard transponder that "turns around" or rebroadcasts incoming messages. We are concerned with this latter subclass and have encircled it in *Figure 33*.

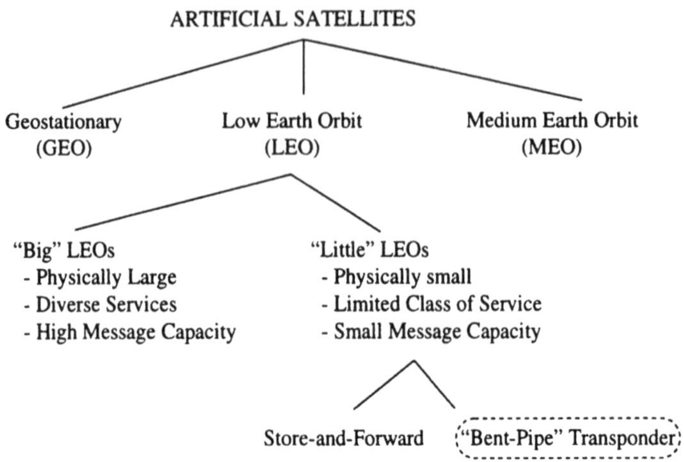


*Figure 33.* The main categories of circular orbit satellite systems.

Our class of interest, the transponding Little LEO, holds promise for inexpensive data transport that may be of significant, if not critical, importance to certain business interests. LEOs have two highly significant advantages over GEOs. First, they are much closer to the Earth and therefore the data round-trip delay is much less than that with a GEO. Second, and often more important, is that a LEO system is one of dynamic geometry as the relative geometrical relationship of the ground-based terminals and the satellite are continuously changing with time. There are many instances where a fixed or long-term non-mobile terminal will not be able to see a GEO but can expect to see a LEO on frequent basis. This is especially true in congested areas such as cities. An article by Akturan and Vogel [5] discloses that in urban Japan, the probability is greater than 50% that an Earth-to-space line of sight will be blocked at an elevation below $25^0$.

Exploitation of the dynamic geometry to capture its inherent advantage has always seemed to be a difficult design issue. The difficulties have been thought to reside in the necessity for a complex protocol controlling access to the transponder capacity. We now examine the idea of using Doppler information to implement flow control for LEO satellite systems. As we have previously noted, the correction for Doppler is a necessity for LEO satellite systems, as the Doppler frequency-shift is significant for these systems. Moreover, for successful reception of information in the outbound channel, terminals are required to estimate and compensate for the Doppler shift. Our new protocol requires only that the terminals keep track of the Doppler frequency-shift versus time characteristic, in addition to compensating for it.

We call the idea embodied in our concept Doppler-Based Multiple Access or DBMA. We use the Doppler frequency shift observed at terminals to control transmissions from them such that the system may function at its capacity limit at all times, i.e., serve as many terminals as possible.

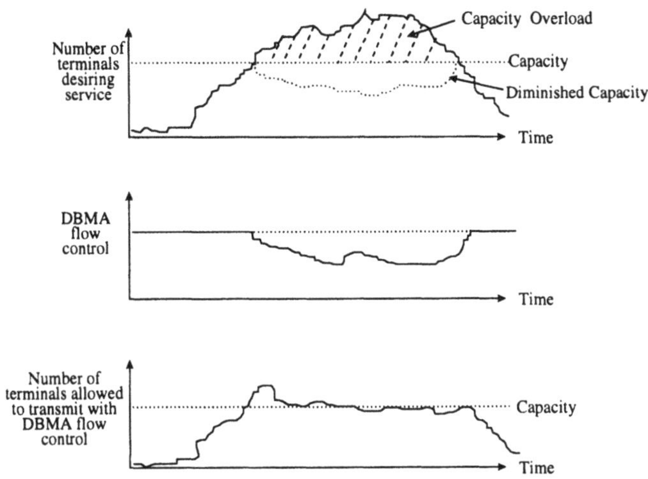


*Figure 34.* A sketch of the function of DBMA.

In a nutshell, DBMA functions as sketched in *Figure 34*. The top graph displays the number of terminals desiring to transmit as the satellite passes over the terminals. This number varies with time due to two factors: (i) the stochastic process of message arrivals at individual terminals, and (ii) the satellite's changing position with respect to the terminals. Terminals in new areas become visible to the satellite and others that were visible are no longer within the visibility footprint of the satellite. For some satellite-terminal geometries, the number of terminals desiring to transmit can be higher than the system capacity and can overload the system, as shown in *Figure 34*. There are two effects of such an overload. First, the terminal transmissions above capacity are surely lost, and second, and perhaps most deleterious to the system, the interference introduced by the simultaneous terminal transmissions above capacity raises background noise levels to existing users and thereby increases the probability of errors in existing terminal transmissions. This overload situation can result in a serious diminution of capacity.

The middle graph is a DBMA flow control, which manages, in a novel way, the number of terminals communicating with the satellite. It is based upon Doppler processing at terminals and is particularly well suited to a Little LEO satellite operating as a "bent-pipe" transponder.

The bottom graph shows the effect of the DBMA flow control on the number of communicating terminals. Note that it is brought to near capacity and thus provides a nearly optimal use of the satellite asset, increasing the *utilized* capacity of the system.

## 2. OVERVIEW OF THE DBMA PROTOCOL

DBMA is a flow control scheme for regulating traffic on the inbound channel. In DBMA, the Earth station specifies a subset of the visibility footprint as a region of eligibility (ROE). Only terminals located in the ROE are permitted to transmit. By varying the size and location of the ROE, effective flow control is achieved on the inbound channel.

DBMA control is a centralized flow control scheme, i.e., the Earth station determines the ROE. This is communicated to the terminals via the outbound channel. The remarkable feature of this method is that the ROE is defined solely by the characteristics of the Doppler frequency-shift versus time function on the outbound channel. The Doppler-time variation observed at terminals is fairly significant because of the low altitude of the satellite's orbit. The Doppler-time curve is a smooth, fast varying "S-curve" due to the rapidly changing geometry between the terminal and satellite.

For illustrative purposes, we consider a configuration comprising a single satellite in a circular orbit. The Earth station is located at San Francisco, and terminals are located in the continental United States. The satellite follows a circular orbit (eccentricity=0) of altitude 1000 km and inclination $53^0$. The revolution period of the satellite is 1.75 hours [9]. This orbit is fairly representative of LEO satellite systems proposed for operation [7]. The cutoff elevation angle for communication is assumed to be $10^0$, i.e., a terminal can communicate with a satellite only if the elevation angle from the terminal to the satellite is greater than or equal to $10^0$. In the remainder of this chapter, when we state that a satellite is visible to a terminal, we mean that the elevation angle from the terminal to the satellite is greater than or equal to $10^0$. The visibility footprint of a satellite is the region on Earth's surface where the elevation angle to the satellite is greater than or equal to $10^0$.

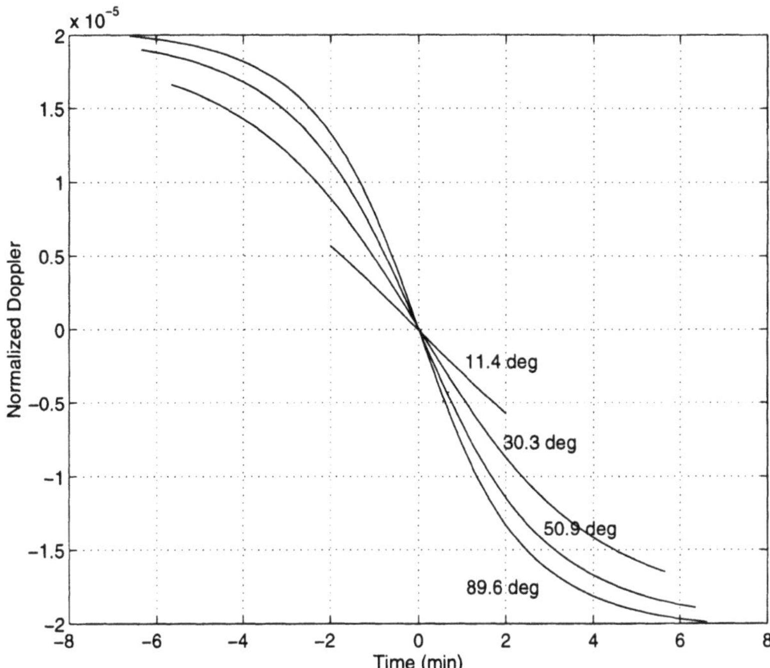


*Figure 35.* Doppler-time S-curve observed at terminals on the outbound downlink channel for maximum elevation angles $11.4^0$, $30.3^0$, $50.9^0$ and $89.6^0$.

The DBMA protocol uses the fact that the Doppler frequency at terminals exhibits a well-behaved variation with time that can be parameterized by the maximum elevation during the visibility duration of the satellite at the terminal. This S-shaped variation is depicted in *Figure 35* for maximum elevation angles ranging from $11.4^0$ to $89.6^0$. Doppler shift is captured in terms of normalized Doppler shift, which is equal to $(v/c)$, where $v$ is the relative velocity of the satellite with respect to the terminal and $c$ is the speed of light. The actual Doppler frequency shift observed at the terminal is $(v/c)*f$ where $f$ is the central frequency of the outbound channel. Time is expressed relative to the zero-Doppler instant. These curves are similar to the ones previously reported in the literature [6]. For a carrier frequency of 150 MHz, the Doppler frequency exhibits noticeable variation, up to 3 kHz, over the satellite visibility time interval. This variation can be measured and tracked in the receiver frequency synchronization circuitry prior to data demodulation

A similar Doppler-time curve is observed at the satellite on the outbound uplink channel (from Earth station to satellite). If the outbound uplink shift is not compensated for, the Doppler shift observed at terminals will be the cumulative effect of the shift in the outbound uplink direction and the outbound downlink direction. However, in most LEO operations, the Earth station monitors and compensates for the Doppler frequency shift in the outbound uplink direction. Hence, the Doppler shift observed at a terminal is due only to the relative geometry between the terminal and the satellite. For the DBMA protocol, it is a *requirement* that the Earth station compensate for the Doppler frequency shift in the outbound uplink direction.

The terminal makes a few Doppler frequency shift measurements. These measurements enable it to determine which Doppler-time curve it is observing. The terminal infers two important parameters from the Doppler-time curve that are used in the DBMA protocol. The first is the maximum elevation angle to the satellite that will be observable at the terminal: $\theta_{max}$. The second is the estimate of the time instant of zero-Doppler: $t_0$. The details of the estimation process are provided in Chapter 2 and in Section 5.

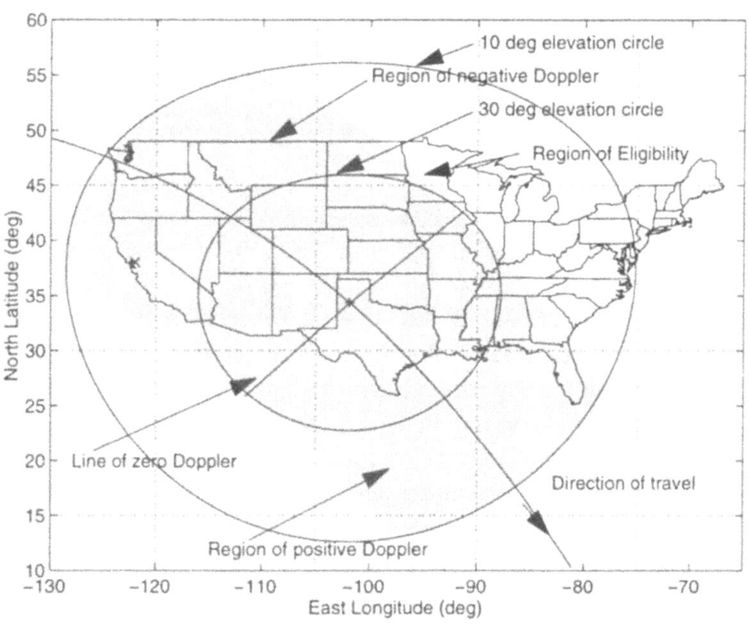


*Figure 36.* ROE for transmission with cutoff maximum elevation angle of $30^0$.

For flow control, the Earth station describes the ROE for transmission in terms of these two parameters. Let us first consider the parameter $\theta_{max}$. In *Figure 36*, the present location of the satellite is over the sub-satellite point shown by a '+' over Texas on the ground trace. The outer circle is the locus of points on the Earth's surface where the elevation angle to the satellite is $10^0$. This is the circumference of the communication visibility region. For all points inside the circle, the elevation angle to the satellite is greater than 10°.

The inner circle is the locus of all points on the Earth where the elevation angle to the satellite is 30°. The edge of the shaded region parallel to the ground trace is the locus of all points on the Earth's surface within the $10^0$ elevation angle circle where the *maximum* elevation angle to the satellite is 30°; the maximum is taken over the visibility duration of the satellite at a terminal. All points in the shaded region will observe maximum elevation angle greater than 30° at some time in their corresponding satellite visibility duration. In the literature, this region is referred to as the 30° swath of the satellite [8].

All terminals in the shaded region observe one of the Doppler S-curves corresponding to maximum elevation angles between $30^0$ and 90° (*Figure 35*). The terminals on the perpendicular to the ground trace at the sub-satellite point observe zero Doppler. The satellite is at its closest approach to these terminals and these terminals observe the maximum elevation angle to the satellite at the present instant. The terminals within the $30^0$ swath behind the zero-Doppler line observe negative instantaneous Doppler frequency shift. These terminals have already observed zero Doppler. Correspondingly, in *Figure 35*, these terminals observe Doppler on the Doppler-time curve to the right of the zero-Doppler instant. The terminals within the $30^0$ swath along the direction of travel of the satellite and ahead of the zero-Doppler observation line observe positive instantaneous Doppler frequency shift. These terminals are yet to observe zero Doppler. Correspondingly, in *Figure 35*, these terminals observe Doppler on the Doppler-time curve to the left of the zero-Doppler instant.

One parameter that the Earth station uses in describing the ROE on the Earth's surface is a cutoff maximum elevation angle $\theta_{max,c}$. Those terminals in the visibility region of the satellite which observe a maximum elevation angle greater than $\theta_{max,c}$ are permitted to transmit. If $\theta_{max,c} = 30^0$, the shaded region of *Figure 36* is the ROE for transmission. The terminals in the 10° visibility region of the satellite, but outside the shaded region are not permitted to transmit.

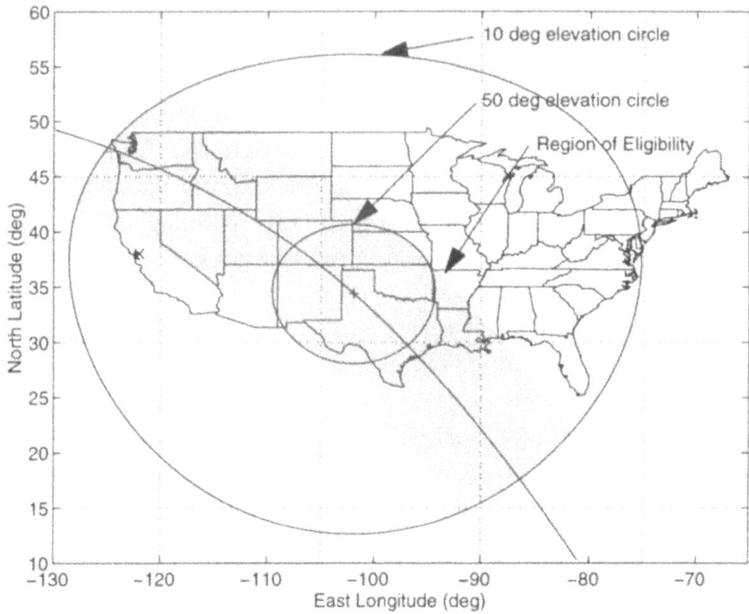


*Figure 37.* ROE for transmission with cutoff maximum elevation angle of $50^0$.

By varying $\theta_{max,c}$ the Earth station controls the contour of the ROE. *Figure 37* shows the ROE for $\theta_{max,c} = 50°$. This region is narrower than the one corresponding to $\theta_{max,c} = 30°$ (*Figure 36*). Hence, $\theta_{max,c}$ determines the width of the ROE. For $\theta_{max,c} = 10°$, the ROE is the entire 10° visibility circle; for $\theta_{max,c} = 90°$ the ROE is the ground trace in the 10° visibility circle.

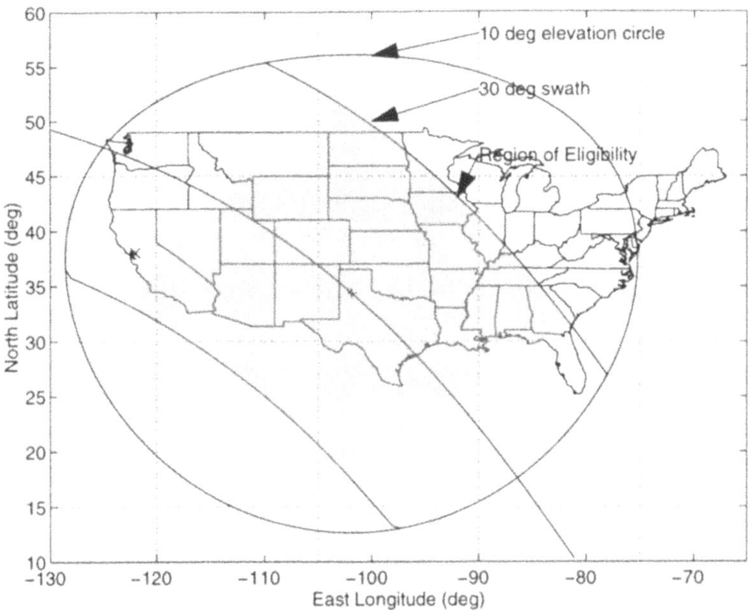


*Figure 38.* ROE corresponding to 8 min [-4,4] interval about the zero Doppler time and cutoff maximum elevation angle $30^0$.

Another parameter the Earth station uses to define the ROE is a time interval about the zero-Doppler instant on the Doppler S-curve. Let us denote this parameter by $t_c$. Those terminals that observe instantaneous Doppler within the time interval $(-t_c, t_c)$ about the zero Doppler time $t_o$ are eligible to transmit. The ROE corresponding to $t_c = 4$ min and $\theta_{max,c} = 30°$ is shown shaded in *Figure 38*. All terminals in the shaded region have either observed zero Doppler during the past 4 minutes or will observe zero Doppler within the next 4 minutes.

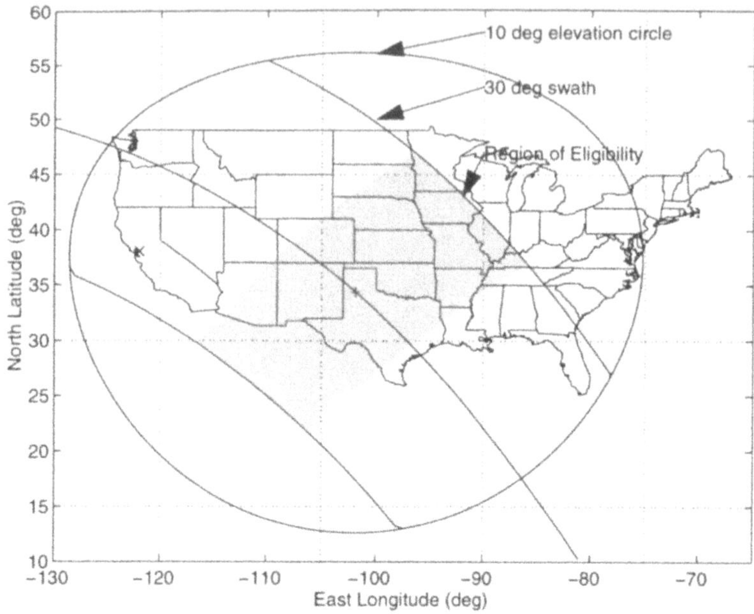


*Figure 39.* ROE corresponding to 4 min [-2,2] interval about the zero Doppler time and $30^0$ swath.

In *Figure 39*, the shaded region corresponds to ROE with $t_c$ =2 min and $\theta_{max,c}$ = 30°. The parameter $t_c$ determines the length of the ROE. Given $\theta_{max,c}$ =30°, for $t_c$ = 0 min, the ROE is a line perpendicular to the ground trace at the sub-satellite point '+'. Terminals on this line observe zero-Doppler at this instant.

Thus, through two parameters, maximum elevation angle $\theta_{max,c}$ and time interval about zero-Doppler, $t_c$, DBMA controls the size of the ROE. This provides a two-axis control of the ROE. By varying the size of the ROE for transmission, DBMA regulates the number of terminals that communicate to the Earth station, thus regulating the load on the inbound channel.

## 3. DBMA PROTOCOL PROCESSES

The DBMA protocol processes are composed of two sub-processes: one at a terminal and one at the Earth station.

### 3.1 At the Terminal

As a satellite comes into common view of a terminal and the Earth station, the terminal determines:

1. the expected maximum elevation of the satellite to the terminal, and
2. the time to the maximum elevation of the satellite.

This information is obtained from the Doppler-time curve observed at the terminal.

The terminal monitors the Earth station outbound link to determine the terminal's eligibility to transmit, should it have a message waiting in the transmit queue. This eligibility is defined by a message from the Earth station in the outbound channel with:

- a lower bound on the maximum elevation of the satellite, and
- limits on a time interval centered at the time of zero Doppler.

If the terminal has a message to transmit, and if it is eligible to transmit during the present satellite pass, the terminal selects a start transmission time at random within the available time window of eligibility.

### 3.2 At the Earth Station

The Earth station monitors the cumulative terminal transmission load on the inbound channel. If this load exceeds the capability of the Earth station, the Earth station reduces the size of ROE for transmissions and broadcasts this restriction. The Earth station controls the ROE by allowing terminals to transmit only if the maximum angle of elevation falls within a tighter set of limits. The Earth station also adjusts the inbound channel load by changing limits of the time window around zero-Doppler instant.

## 4. SIMULATION RESULTS

We illustrate the effectiveness of DBMA through simulations. The simulation assumes a single satellite in a circular orbit of altitude 1000 km and orbit inclination $53^0$. Terminals are modeled as point sources of traffic located in the continental United States. For our simulation, we assumed 10,000 terminals uniformly distributed over a rectangular area between the latitudes of 30° N and 50° N, and longitudes -125° E and -75° E, which serves as an approximation of the geographical extent of the continental US. Terminals communicate with the Earth station through the satellite when the satellite is visible (greater than $10^0$ elevation angle) to *both* the terminal and Earth station.

Load on the inbound channel, in our simulation, is measured by the number of terminals that can communicate to the Earth station. We have used this simple definition to introduce and illustrate the operation of DBMA flow control. As discussed previously, DBMA controls traffic on the network by changing the size of the ROE for transmission. This regulates the load on the network irrespective of whether load is measured in terms of number of nodes transmitting or number of messages per unit time.

For the results provided here, we have assumed that terminals are able to exactly determine the correct Doppler-time curve they are observing. Hence, they make no errors in estimating the maximum elevation angle to the satellite and the time to zero-Doppler. Also, we have ignored the latency between the transmission of the two parameters $\theta_{max,c}$ and $t_c$ and its reception by terminals in the visibility footprint of the satellite.

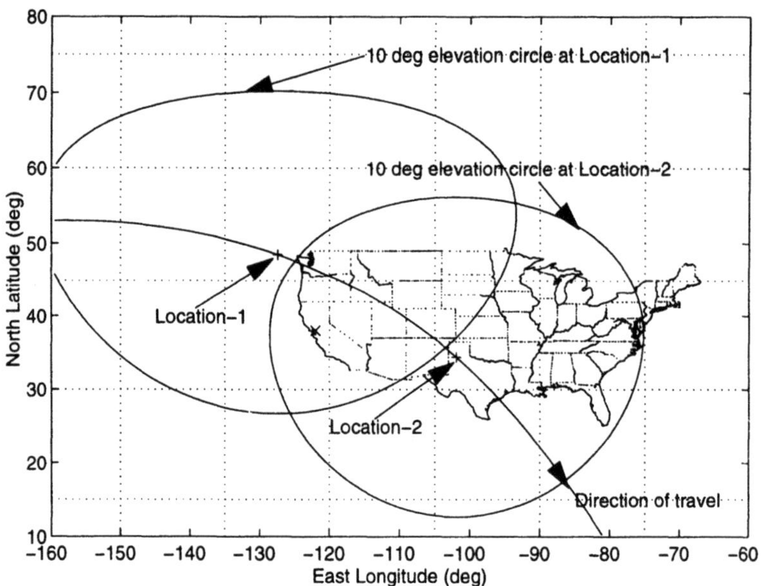


*Figure 40.* $10^0$ visibility region of satellite for two locations of the satellite separated in time by 7.2 minutes.

To appreciate the dynamics of the load on the inbound channel as the location of satellite changes, consider *Figure 40*. There we show a segment of the ground trace along with 10° visibility regions for two locations of the satellite separated in time by 7.2 minutes. These locations are marked by '+' on the ground trace. The location of the Earth station is represented in the figure by an 'x' in San Francisco. The load on the channel varies dynamically as new regions on Earth become visible to the satellite while other regions that were visible are no longer within the visibility footprint of the satellite. This is illustrated in *Figure 41*, which plots the load on the inbound channel with time for one pass of the satellite over the US. Time is expressed in minutes from the start of the simulation. The traffic increases from 1000 terminals to about 9000 terminals as more areas of the US are covered by the $10^0$ visibility footprint of the satellite. The traffic drops off to zero suddenly at the end of the pass as the satellite loses visibility to the Earth station. The capacity of the system is assumed to be fixed at 6000 terminals.

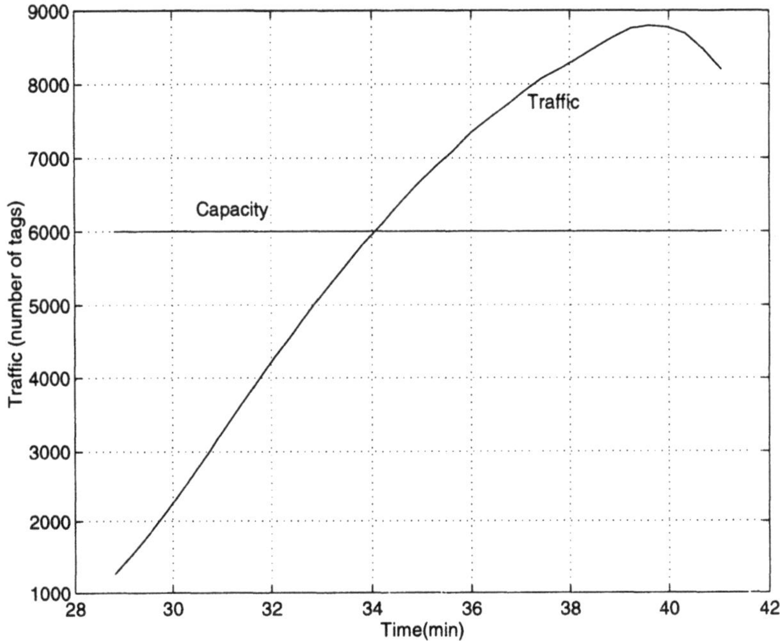


*Figure 41*. Traffic variation during a single pass of the satellite.

The algorithm at the Earth station for determining $\theta_{max,c}$ and $t_c$ is as follows: If traffic from the ROE is greater than the capacity, (Step 1) increase $\theta_{max,c}$ by $\Delta\theta$ (=$5^0$) and check if the traffic is below capacity; if not, (Step 2) reduce $t_c$ by $\Delta t_c$ (=30 sec) and check if traffic is below capacity. Repeat steps 1 and 2 until the traffic is just below capacity. The initial condition is to let the ROE be the entire $10^0$ visibility region ($\theta_{max,c} = 10^0$ and $t_c = 7$ min).

Traffic is measured by counting the number of terminals within the ROE. The simulation is advanced every 21.6 seconds (4000 samples in a 24 hour day), the new location of the satellite generated, and the DBMA protocol applied.

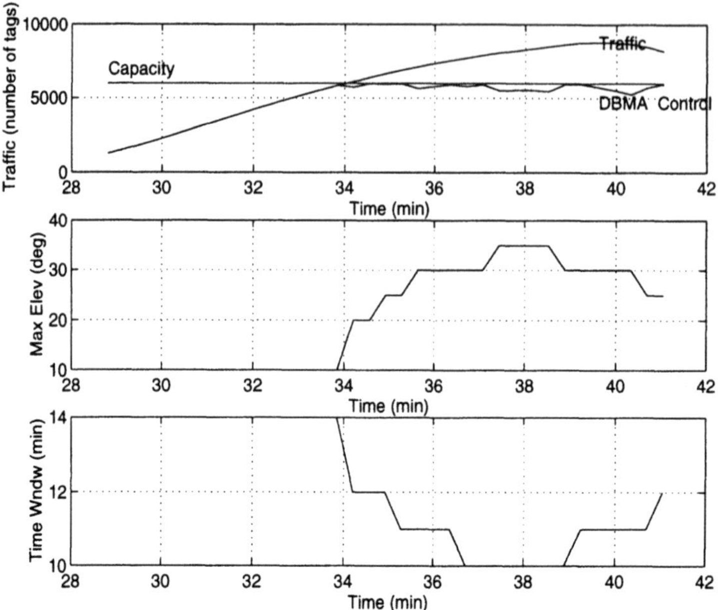


*Figure 42.* Result of simulation of DBMA protocol for flow control, pass A.

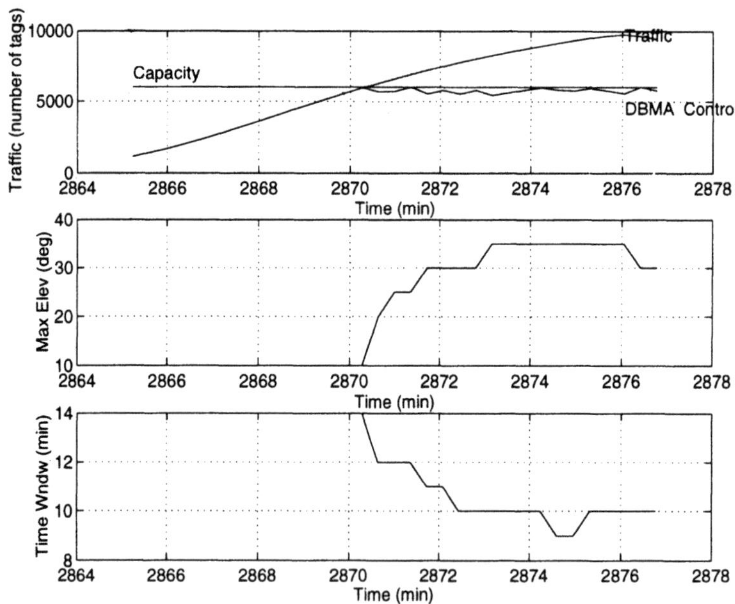


*Figure 43.* Result of simulation of DBMA protocol for flow control, pass B.

*Figure 42* and *Figure 43* show the result of applying the DBMA protocol for two different passes of the satellite over the continental US. Each figure consists of three plots. The first plot has three curves. The first curve depicts the uncontrolled traffic on the inbound channel. The second curve shows the capacity of the inbound link. The third curve is a plot of the load on the inbound channel as a result of DBMA. The second and the third plots show the time variations of the control parameters $\theta_{max,c}$ and $t_c$ respectively.

From these two figures, we observe that the DBMA protocol is very effective in throttling the load on the inbound channel at or below capacity. When the load on the channel is below the rated capacity of the channel, all terminals in the visibility footprint are permitted to transmit, i.e., the ROE is the $10^0$ visibility footprint. When traffic goes above the rated capacity, DBMA modifies the ROE to maintain the load at its rated capacity. The control algorithm at the Earth station does not exhibit oscillations in the value of the two control parameters with time.

# 5. DOPPLER CURVE ESTIMATION

The prediction of the maximum elevation angle $\theta_{max}$ and zero-Doppler time $t_0$ using Doppler frequency measurements was provided in Chapter 2 based on the analytical expression for the Doppler S-curve. In this section, we provide a simpler scheme to predict these quantities based on curve-fitting of the Doppler S-curve.

Careful inspection of *Figure 35* shows that if we consider transmission times up to $t_0$, the Doppler-time characteristics can be approximated by a quadratic functional dependence. We show a sample of our quadratic Doppler curve fitting results in *Figure 44* for a maximum elevation angle of $39.4^0$. The estimate was computed using three Doppler frequency measurements during the first 3 minutes of satellite visibility. It is noted that for small elevation angles (less than 25 degrees), the Doppler-time characteristic is linear.

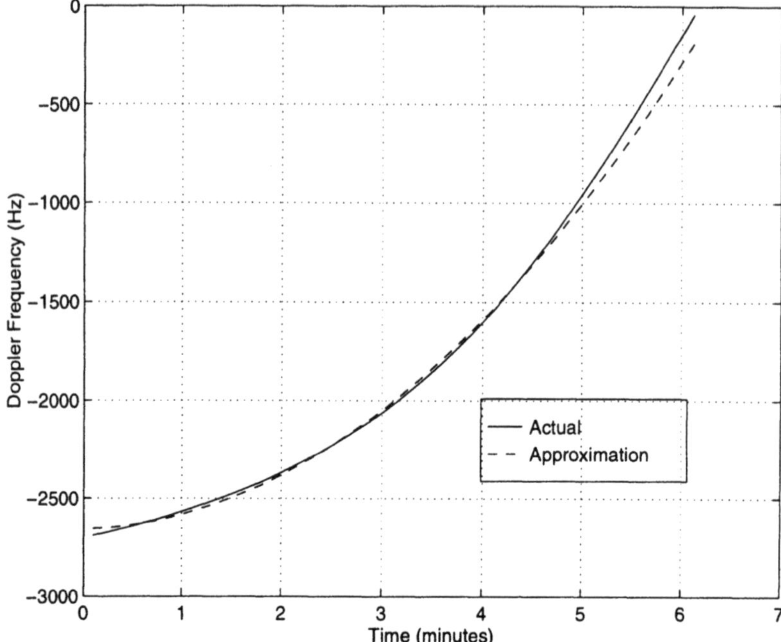


*Figure 44.* Quadratic curve fitting to the Doppler S-curve for $39.4^0$ maximum elevation angle.

*Figure 45* shows the variation of the mean square estimation error (in dB) between the actual and estimated Doppler frequency. In *Figure 46*, we have plotted the ideal value of $t_0$ together with its estimated value (using quadratic curve fitting) as a function of maximum elevation angle. It can be seen from the figures that the maximum error in estimating the zero-Doppler instant is less than 1.5 minutes.

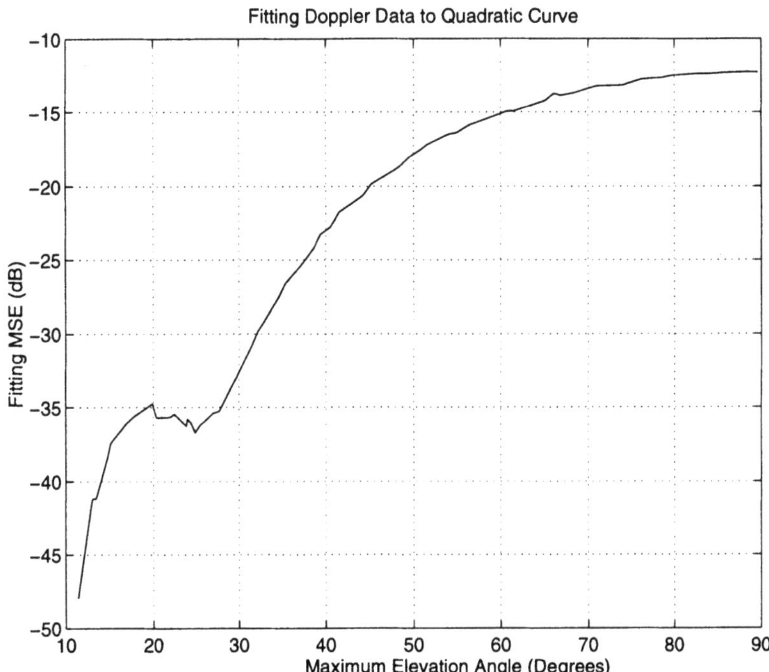


*Figure 45.* Mean square error for quadratic curve fitting for Doppler S-curve.

Fitting accuracy for higher maximum elevation angles can be improved by using more Doppler measurements and using a higher-order polynomial fit. Another means for improving fitting accuracy is to use Doppler rate measurements in conjunction with the direct Doppler data, as in [10] and in Chapter 2. As shown in *Figure 47*, the Doppler rate of change decreases appreciably as the satellite approaches the terminal, and it reaches a minimum at $t_0$.

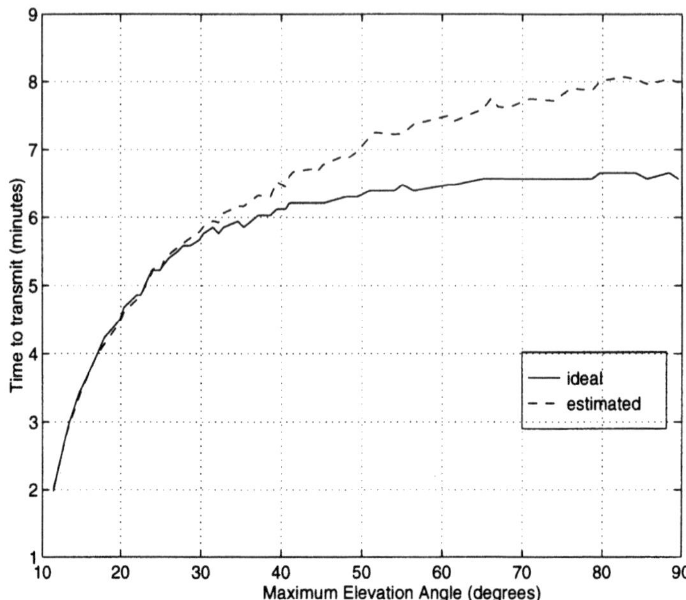


*Figure 46.* Estimation of zero-Doppler time.

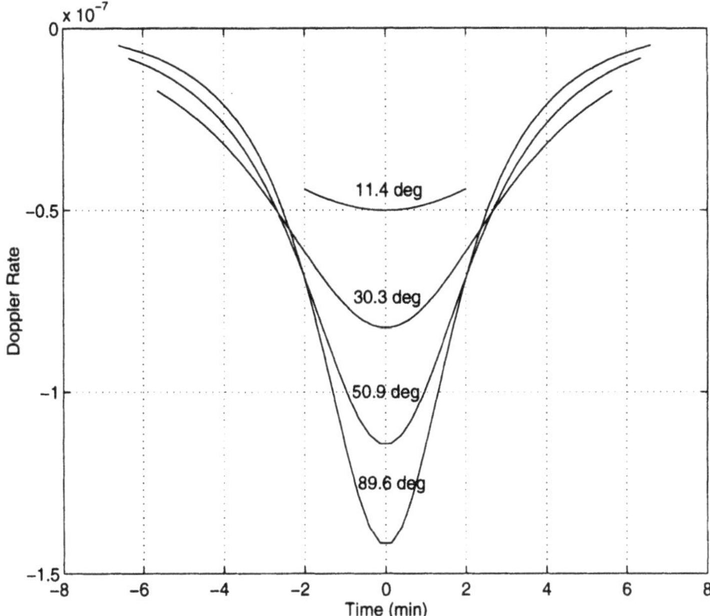


*Figure 47.* Rate of change of Doppler vs. time for maximum elevation angles $11.4^0$, $30.3^0$, $50.9^0$ and $89.6^0$.

# REFERENCES

[1] J.E. Hershey, I. Ali, N. Al-Dhahir, G. J. Saulnier, and R. Nelson, 'Method and apparatus for Doppler based multiple access communication control,' Patent filed (1996).

[2] A. H. Ballard, 'Rosette Constellations of Earth Satellites,' *IEEE Transactions on Aerospace and Electronic Systems*, Vol. AES-16, No. 5, p. 656-673 (1980).

[3] J. G. Walker, 'Continuous whole Earth coverage by circular orbit satellite patterns,' *Royal Aircraft Establishment, Tech, Report 77044* (UDC 629. 195:527); available through DDC, AD-A044593, unclassified (1977).

[4] J. Radzik, and G. Maral, 'A methodology for rapidly evaluating the performance of some low Earth orbit satellite systems,' *IEEE Journal of Selected Areas in Communications*, Vol. 13, No. 2, p. 301-309 (1995).

[5] R. Akturan and W.J. Vogel, 'Elevation angle dependence of fading for satellite PCS in urban areas,' *Electronic Letters*, Vol. 31 No. 25, p. 2156-2157 (1995).

[6] M. Katayama, A. Ogawa, and N. Morinaga, 'Carrier Synchronization Under Doppler Shift of the Nongeostationary satellite communication system,' *Proc. of ICCS/ISITA '92*, p. 466-470 (1992).

[7] B. Gerding, 'Odyssey: Going global with wireless personal communications,' *Wireless Design and Development*, p. 21-22 (1992).

[8] D.C. Beste, 'Design of satellite constellations for optimal continuous coverage,' *IEEE Tranasctions on Aerospace Electronics*, Vol. AES-14, p. 466-473 (1978).

[9] W.L. Pritchard, H.G. Suyderhoud and R.A. Nelson, *Satellite Communication Systems Engineering*, Prentice Hall, Englewood Cliffs, New Jersey, (1993).
[10] I. Ali, N. Al-Dhahir, and J. E. Hershey, "Doppler Characterization for LEO Satellites," *IEEE Transactions on Communications*, Vol. 46, No. 3, March 1998, p. 309-313.

# Chapter 6

# Doppler for Power Control

In this chapter, we introduce two schemes for uplink power control based on the Doppler S-curve observed at mobile terminals. In the first scheme, termed Doppler Based Transmit Power Control (DBTPOWC), terminals estimate their distance from the satellite using the Doppler S-curve and modify their transmitted power to compensate for the path loss differential to the satellite. In the second scheme, termed Doppler Based Transmit Permission Control (DBTPERMC), the Earth station permits only those terminals to transmit whose distance from the satellite is within a specified range. The regions of eligibility (ROE) in DBTPERMC are regions between concentric ellipses centered at the sub-satellite point, instead of the parallelogram regions of DBMA.

## 1. INTRODUCTION

Because of their simplicity and low complexity as multiple-access schemes, code division multiple-access (CDMA) and spread-ALOHA have been proposed as multiple-access schemes on the uplink channel in LEO satellite systems [2]. These schemes require minimal coordination among transmitting mobile terminals, and the channel throughput performance of these schemes degrades gracefully as the load on the channel increases. One of the key disadvantages of these schemes is the requirement for power control by mobile terminals: for optimal performance, the received power levels at the satellite from the transmitting terminals should be approximately the same. For LEO satellite systems, this problem is further exacerbated by the dynamic geometry between satellite and mobile terminals.

In this chapter, we introduce two effective schemes for power control on the uplink channel of LEO satellite systems. Both of these schemes are based on the Doppler observed by mobile terminals on the downlink channel. For LEO satellite systems, this Doppler is significant and is a smooth, S shaped curve [4]. For effectively decoding information on the downlink channel, mobile terminals must estimate and compensate for this Doppler. Hence, the Doppler information is already available at mobile terminals.

Transmit power control schemes reported in the literature have been broadly classified into two categories [6]: *open-loop* power control, in which the mobile terminal monitors a pilot in the downlink channel and modifies its transmit power accordingly, and *feedback-loop* power control, in which messages in the downlink channel instruct the terminal to transmit at the desired power level. The schemes proposed in this chapter are open-loop power-control schemes.

Transmit permission control as a means for power control by reducing interference due to excessive number of simultaneous transmissions was independently introduced in [1] and [3] for LEO satellite systems. In [1], a pilot signal transmitted in the downlink channel is used by mobile terminals to determine their distance from the satellite. The Earth station permits only those mobile terminals to transmit whose distance from the satellite is less than a specified value. Geographically, this amounts to specifying a region of eligibility (ROE) on the ground that is a circle with radius smaller than that of the visibility footprint [1]. In [3], the ROEs are parallelograms parallel to the ground trace of the satellite and centered at the sub-satellite point. The ROEs in [3] were specified in terms of the Doppler-time curve observed by mobile terminals.

The key advantages of the two power control schemes proposed here for LEO satellite systems, with respect to the open-loop power control and Jamalipour's transmit permission control scheme [1], is that the schemes proposed here accomplish power control with existing Doppler information at mobile terminals, without requiring additional information such as a pilot signal in the downlink channel. However, these schemes are specifically for non-fading channels, and only compensate for path length variations. The non-fading assumption is a proper simplification for high elevation angles in LEO satellite systems [2, pg. 209]. For fading channels, the Doppler based power control schemes proposed here can be supplemented with either open-loop or feedback-loop power control schemes that compensate for the fast fading characteristics of the channel. In this case, the Doppler based power control schemes compensate for the relatively slow variation in distance to the satellite.

## 2. DOPPLER CHARACTERIZATION

For LEO satellites, the Doppler frequency at terminals exhibits a well-behaved variation with time that can be characterized by the maximum elevation angle from the terminal to the satellite during the visibility window. This S-shaped variation is depicted in *Figure 48* for maximum elevation angles ranging from $11.4^0$ to $90^0$ degrees for a terminal located at latitude $39^0$ *N* and longitude $77^0$ *W*. The satellite follows a circular orbit (eccentricity=0) of altitude 1000 km and inclination $53^0$. The minimum elevation angle for visibility is assumed to be $10^0$. Doppler information is captured in terms of normalized Doppler shift, which is equal to $(v/c)$, where $v$ is the relative velocity of the satellite with respect to the terminal, and $c$ is the speed of light. Time is expressed relative to the zero-Doppler instant. The zero-Doppler instant is the time during the visibility window at which the elevation angle from the terminal to the satellite is at its maximum value and the satellite is at its closest approach to the terminal. The Doppler frequency shift is shown only for the visibility duration of the satellite at the terminal; the visibility duration increases as the maximum elevation angle to the satellite increases.

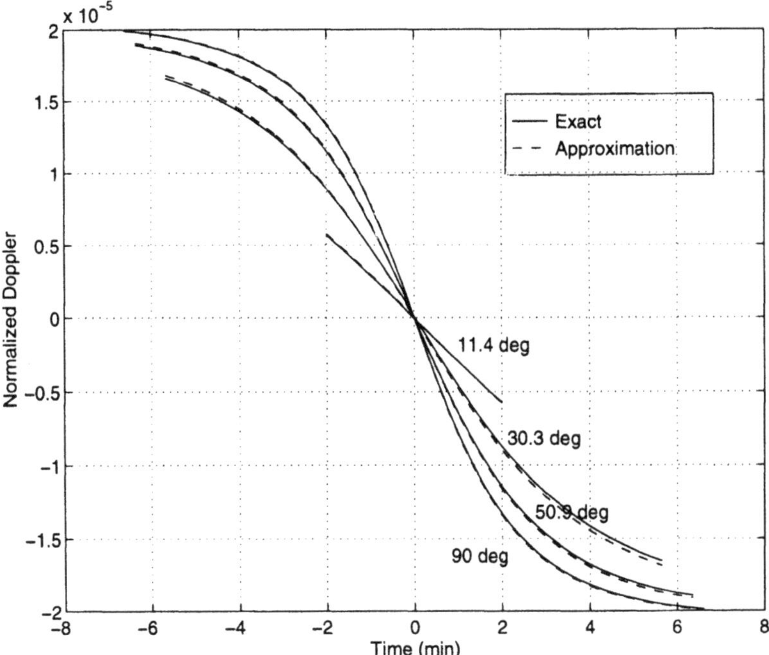


*Figure 48.* Actual and approximate Doppler-time S-curve for maximum elevation angles $11.4^0$, $30.3^0$, $50.9^0$ and $90^0$.

In [4], we developed analytic approximations to the Doppler-time curve and we outlined a simple algorithm by which a mobile terminal determines the maximum elevation angle to the satellite, $\theta_{max}$, and the zero-Doppler instant, $t_0$, based on two Doppler and-Doppler rate measurements taken at the beginning of the visibility window of the satellite. The instantaneous elevation angle, $\theta(t)$, from a mobile terminal to a satellite is given by [5, Equation (3-4)]

$$\cos\theta(t) = \frac{r\sin\gamma(t)}{\sqrt{r_E^2 + r^2 - 2r_E r\cos\gamma(t)}} \qquad (1)$$

where

$r_E$ radius of the Earth,

$r$ radius of the satellite's orbit,

$\gamma(t)$ central angle between the point on the Earth and the sub-satellite point. This is given by [4, Equation (10)], i.e., $\cos\gamma(t) = \cos\omega_F(t - t_0)\cos\gamma(t_0)$ where $\omega_F$ is the angular velocity of the satellite in the ECF frame approximated by [4, Equation (9)] and $\gamma(t_0)$ is given by [4, Equation (4)].

The distance to the satellite, $d$, is a function of the elevation angle to the satellite and is given by [5, Equation (3-7)]

$$d = \sqrt{r^2 - (r_E\cos\theta)^2} - r_E\sin\theta \qquad (2)$$

In *Figure 49* we plot the instantaneous elevation angle with respect to time from the zero-Doppler instant, for different values of $\theta_{max}$, and for the satellite orbit parameters used for *Figure 48*. Thus, using the Doppler-time estimation algorithm and the above equations, each mobile terminal determines its distance to the satellite.

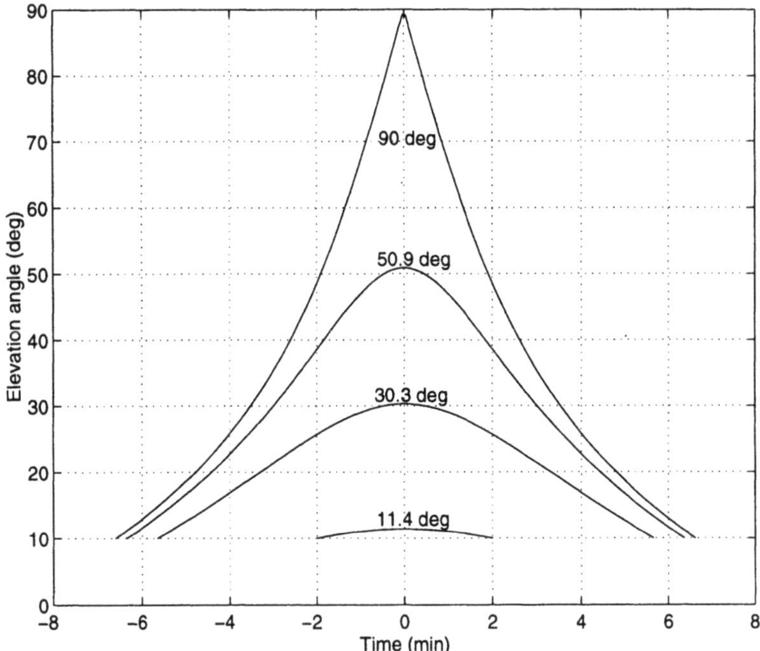


*Figure 49.* Elevation angle as a function of time for different maximum elevation angles $11.4^0$, $30.3^0$, $50.9^0$ and $90^0$.

## 3. DOPPLER BASED TRANSMIT POWER CONTROL (DBTPOWC)

Let the desired received power level at the satellite from mobile terminals be $S$. In a non-fading channel, the transmitted power of the $i$-th user should be [1]

$$T_i(t) = \kappa \ S \ d_i^2(t) \tag{3}$$

where $\kappa$ is constant and $d_i$ is the distance of the $i$-th user from the satellite. As stated in the previous section, the mobile terminal determines its distance to the satellite from the Doppler-time curve and then transmits at the desired level.

# 4. DOPPLER BASED TRANSMIT PERMISSION CONTROL (DBTPERMC)

In DBTPermC, the Earth station specifies an ROE on the ground such that transmissions are allowed only from mobile terminals within the ROE. The received power from these transmissions is within a specified range. The ROEs are specified such that the received power at the satellite from all the permitted mobiles is within a narrow range. From Equation (3), this can be achieved by restricting the permitted mobiles to be at approximately the same distance from the satellite. Since terminals with equal elevation angle to the satellite are at the same distance from the satellite, the Earth station specifies ROE in terms of a permitted range in the elevation angle. The ROEs are now circular bands on the Earth's surface centered at the sub-satellite point. We show the ROEs for two ranges of permitted elevation angle ($30^0$,$40^0$) and ($60^0$,$70^0$) in *Figure 50.* Mobile terminals determine their instantaneous elevation angle from the Doppler-time curves, and transmit only if their elevation angles are within the specified range.

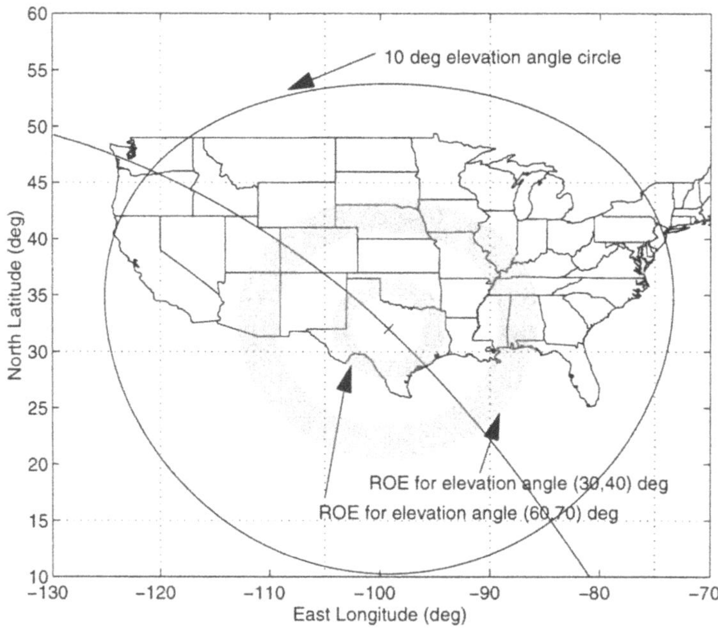


*Figure 50.* Region of eligibility (ROE) for elevation angle ranges ($30^0$,$40^0$) and ($60^0$,$70^0$).

In DBTPermC, the mobile terminals may or may not use active transmit power control. Using active transmit power control, such as DBTPowC, would further improve performance.

## REFERENCES

[1] A. Jamalipour, et al., "Transmit Permission Control on Spread Aloha Packets in LEO Satellite Systems," *IEEE Journal of Selected Areas in Communications*, Vol. 14, No. 9, pp. 1748-1757, 1996.

[2] A. Jamalipour, *Low Earth Orbital Satellites for Personal Communication Networks*, Artech House, Norwood, MA, 1998.

[3] I. Ali, N. Al-Dhahir, J.E. Hershey, G.J. Saulnier, and R. Nelson, "Doppler as a New Dimension for Multiple-access in LEO Satellite Systems," *International Journal of Satellite Communications*, Vol. 15 No. 6, Nov-Dec 1997, p. 269-279.

[4] I. Ali, N. Al-Dhahir, and J. E. Hershey, "Doppler Characterization for LEO Satellites," *IEEE Transactions on Communications*, Vol. 46, No. 3, March 1998, p. 309-313.

[5] W.L. Pritchard, H.G. Suyderhoud and R.A. Nelson, *Satellite Communication Systems Engineering*, Prentice Hall, 1993.

[6] T. Rappaport, *Wireless Communications: Principles and Practice*, Prentice-Hall Inc., NJ, 1996.

# Chapter 7

# DBMA Simulation Software

To aid the reader in the visualization of LEO satellite orbit geometry and dynamics of the DBMA protocol, we have provided a small but instructive set of MATLAB® simulation routines. This chapter, like the software, is written to serve two types of users. For the busy reader who wishes simply to run the simulations without particular interest in how they work, we provide immediate instructions on how to load and use a set of demonstration functions that are driven by a simple graphical user interface (GUI). For the more interested reader, we describe the architecture of the package and the mathematical algorithms implemented. We end by providing a formal function reference that details the usage of each routine, enabling those who might wish to advance the material in this book the benefit of a few useful tools to aid the work.

## 1. LOADING AND USING THE DEMO SOFTWARE

The complete set of routines is available on CD-ROM provided with the book. Alternatively, the software and any future updates can be accessed via the MathWorks Web site. Instructions for download are

Web: `ftp://ftp.mathworks.com/pub/books/bonanni`

® MATLAB is a registered trademark of The MathWorks, Inc.
For MATLAB product information, please contact: The MathWorks, Inc., 3 Apple Hill Drive, Natick, MA, 01760-2098, USA. Tel: 508-647-7000. Fax: 508-647-7101. E-mail: info@mathworks.com. Web: www.mathworks.com.

Unix login:
```
ftp ftp.mathworks.com
Name: anonymous
Guest login ok, send your complete e-mail address
Password: (type in e-mail address)
cd /pub/books/bonanni
```

The routines have been tested with Versions 5.3.1, 6.0, and 6.1 of MATLAB.

To install the software, simply copy all the provided files to a convenient folder. Upon startup of MATLAB, use the `path` command to ensure that the selected folder is included in the search path. Then enter a demo command (`demo1`, `demo2`, `demo3`, ...) to bring up a GUI from which an animation can be launched.

The following animations are included in the initial release:

- `demo1` - **Satellite ground track animation.** This demo animates the ground track of a typical LEO satellite. The chosen trajectory is an inclined circular orbit at 1000 km altitude.
- `demo2` - **Visibility-based coverage region animation.** This demo displays and animates the visibility-based coverage region of a typical LEO satellite. Visibility from points on the Earth's surface is established if the satellite appears above a given elevation angle in the sky. The satellite in this demo follows an inclined circular orbit at 1000 km altitude.
- `demo3` - **DBMA-based coverage region animation.** This demo displays and animates the DBMA-based coverage region of a typical LEO satellite. The "region of eligibility" for DBMA coverage is symmetric about the sub-satellite point and is given by the intersection of three larger regions:
  - (1) Visibility cone around the sub-satellite point – the region in which the elevation to the satellite from the ground exceeds a given angle. Nodes may transmit at a given time only if the satellite is above this elevation.
  - (2) Orbital swath – the region defined by a lower bound to the maximum elevation angle to the satellite. Only nodes that have observed, or will observe, an elevation angle greater than the given value upon closest passage of the satellite during the current orbital cycle are permitted to transmit.
  - (3) Orbital time window – the region observing closest passage of the satellite within a given time window. Only nodes that have observed (will observe) maximum

elevation within this interval from the given time are permitted to transmit.

The satellite in this demo follows an inclined circular orbit at 1000 km altitude.

# 2. OVERVIEW OF ROUTINES

The demos described above are built on a platform of satellite oriented routines and some supporting math functions that supplement the basic MATLAB command set. The most direct reliance is on two high-level routines, `walker` and `dbmacover`, which compute the satellite orbits and the DBMA coverage regions displayed dynamically in the animations. Function `walker` generates orbit trajectories for a Walker satellite constellation, which describes a pattern of identical circular orbits regularly spaced about a series of planes at a fixed inclination. Function `dbmacover` computes the geographic "region of eligibility" defined by the DBMA protocol of Chapter 5, given parameters specifying the visibility cone, the orbital swath, and the orbital time window.

The satellite oriented support functions on which these high-level routines are based are next listed and described:

- `arcangle` – Calculates the angular distance (central angle) between two terrestrial surface points specified by latitude and longitude.
- `drawmap` – Draws a map using a rectangular grid projection (latitude versus longitude). A *map* is defined as a sequence of contiguous latitude-longitude pairs delimited by "pen-up" indications. Example maps are provided in the MAT-file `maps.mat`. Included are maps representing Earth land-water boundaries, U.S. state borders, and a grid constructed from parallels of latitude and meridians of longitude.
- `eci2ecf2` – Transforms a position/velocity trajectory from Earth-centered-inertial (ECI) to Earth-centered-fixed (ECF) coordinates.
- `greatarc` – Computes a latitude-longitude sequence representing the great circle arc connecting two terrestrial surface points.
- `grnwich` – Calculates the Greenwich right ascension for a given Julian date and time. This is used to compensate for Earth rotation in transformations between ECI and ECF coordinates.
- `intreg` – Computes a latitude-longitude sequence representing the intersection of two geographic regions, themselves defined by latitude-longitude sequences.

- `kepl2eci` - Transforms Keplerian to ECI coordinates. Keplerian coordinates are convenient for specification of elliptical orbits; conversion to ECI enables Cartesian representation of position and velocity.
- `lonlat` - Calculates longitude, latitude, and range from a Cartesian position specification (ECI or ECF). Opposite of `posllr`.
- `orbitper` - Calculates the orbital period as a function of semi-major axis for satellites in orbit about Earth.
- `perimvis` - Computes a latitude-longitude sequence describing the perimeter of the region on Earth's surface visible from a given position in space. Visibility is defined by the criterion that the elevation to the satellite from the ground exceeds a given angle.
- `posllr` - Calculates Cartestian position (ECI or ECF) given longitude, latitude, and range. Opposite of `lonlat`.
- `str2jt` - Converts a date-time string specification to a real-valued Julian time in days, suitable for use in astronomical formulas.
- `swath` - Generates a latitude-longitude sequence defining the swath of visibility for an orbit. Visibility from a given ground point is defined by the criterion that the maximum elevation reached by the satellite on the current pass exceeds a given angle.
- `ucompass` - Calculates unit vectors defining local bearings (East, North, and Zenith) for a given latitude and longitude on Earth.

Additionally, the satellite routines make use of the following mathematical support functions:

- `pvdeg` - Principal value in degrees. Converts angles outside the range $0<\theta<360$ degrees to the equivalent angle in that range.
- `pvdegs` - Symmetric principal value in degrees. Converts angles outside the range $-180<\theta<180$ degrees to the equivalent angle in that range.
- `pvrad` - Principal value in radians. Converts angles outside the range $0<\theta<2\pi$ radians to the equivalent angle in that range.
- `pvrads` - Symmetric principal value in radians. Converts angles outside the range $-\pi<\theta<\pi$ radians to the equivalent angle in that range.
- `rot3x` - Computes the 3x3 matrix representing a rotation about the x-axis by a given angle.
- `rot3y` - Computes the 3x3 matrix representing a rotation about the y-axis by a given angle.

- `rot3z` - Computes the 3x3 matrix representing a rotation about the z-axis by a given angle.
- `rotate3x` - Rotates a 3-space trajectory about the x-axis.
- `rotate3y` - Rotates a 3-space trajectory about the y-axis.
- `rotate3z` - Rotates a 3-space trajectory about the z-axis.

# 3. FUNCTION REFERENCE

---

```
ARCANGLE - Angular distance between surface points.
angle = arcangle(elon1,nlat1,elon2,nlat2)

Calculates the angular distance between surface points
(elon1,nlat1) and (elon2,nlat2), along the great arc
connecting the points.  Inputs 'elon1' and 'elon2' are
in east longitude degrees and 'nlat1' and 'nlat2' are in
north latitude degrees.  These may be scalars or column
vectors of uniform length.  Output 'angle' (scalar or
vector, matching the inputs) is returned in degrees.

P.G. Bonanni
6/29/00
```

---

```
DBMACOVER - Coverage region using DBMA protocol.
[elon,nlat] =
dbmacover(xECF,vECF,index,dt,elev1,elev2,tmax)

Calculates a longitude and latitude sequence (elon,nlat)
defining the boundary of the region within which tags
are allowed to communicate by the DBMA protocol.  This
"region of eligibility," computed for a specific instant
in time, is symmetric about the sub-satellite point and
is given by the intersection of three larger regions:

1) Visibility cone around the sub-satellite point - the
   region in which the elevation to the satellite from
   the ground exceeds a given angle, specified by
   'elev1' in degrees.  Nodes may transmit only if the
   satellite is above this elevation at the current
   time.
2) Orbital swath - the region defined by a lower bound
   to the maximum elevation angle to the satellite,
   specified by 'elev2' in degrees.  Only nodes that
   have observed, or will observe, an elevation angle
```

```
   greater than this value upon closest passage of the
   satellite during the current orbital cycle are
   permitted to transmit.
3) Orbital time window - the region observing closest
   passage of the satellite within a given time window,
   whose half width is specified by 'tmax' in seconds.
   Only nodes that have observed (or will observe)
   maximum elevation within +/- this interval from the
   current time are permitted to transmit.

Parameters:
  xECF - Earth-centered-fixed satellite location [x,y,z]
         in km
  vECF - Earth-centered-fixed satellite velocity
         [vx,vy,vz] in km/sec
  index- index into xECF (and vECF) defining the current
         time
  dt   - time between orbit samples, in sec
  elev1- minimum current visibility angle, in degrees
  elev2- minimum visibility at closest passage, in
         degrees
  tmax - maximum time preceding/following closest
         passage, in sec

NOTE: A negative value for 'tmax' specifies use of the
full time window during which the visibility and maximum
elevation criteria are met.

Units for (elon,nlat) are east longitude degrees and
north latitude degrees, respectively.

Irfan Ali / P.G. Bonanni
7/10/00
```

---

```
DEMO1 - Satellite ground track animation.
demo1(action)

This demo animates the ground track of a typical LEO
satellite.  The chosen trajectory is an inclined
circular orbit at 1000 km altitude.

Possible button actions:
'initialize' - initialize UI and graphics
'start'      - start animation
'stop'       - stop animation
'info'       - display help info
'close'      - close graphics window
```

```
P.G. Bonanni / Irfan Ali  7/17/00
```

---

```
DEMO2 - Visibility-based coverage region animation.
demo2(action)

This demo displays and animates the visibility-based
coverage region of a typical LEO satellite.  Visibility
from points on the Earth's surface is established if the
satellite appears above a given elevation angle in the
sky.  The satellite in this demo follows an inclined
circular orbit at 1000 km altitude.

Possible button actions:
'initialize' - initialize UI and graphics
'start'      - start animation
'stop'       - stop animation
'info'       - display help info
'close'      - close graphics window

P.G. Bonanni / Irfan Ali  7/18/00
```

---

```
DEMO3 - DBMA-based coverage region animation.
demo3(action)

This demo displays and animates the DBMA-based coverage
region of a typical LEO satellite.  The "region of
eligibility" for DBMA coverage is symmetric about the
sub-satellite point and is given by the intersection of
three larger regions:

1) Visibility cone around the sub-satellite point - the
   region in which the elevation to the satellite from
   the ground exceeds a given angle, given by 'elev1' in
   degrees.  Nodes may transmit at a given time only if
   the satellite is above this elevation.
2) Orbital swath - the region defined by a lower bound
   to the maximum elevation angle to the satellite,
   given by 'elev2' in degrees.  Only nodes that have
   observed, or will observe, an elevation angle greater
   than this value upon closest passage of the satellite
   during the current orbital cycle are permitted to
   transmit.
3) Orbital time window - the region observing closest
   passage of the satellite within a given time window,
   given by 'tmax' in seconds.  Only nodes that have
```

```
   observed (will observe) maximum elevation within this
   interval from the given time are permitted to
   transmit. (NOTE: A negative value for 'tmax'
   specifies use of the full time window during which
   the visibility criteria above are met.)

The satellite in this demo follows an inclined circular
orbit at 1000 km altitude.

Possible button actions:
'initialize' - initialize UI and graphics
'start'      - start animation
'stop'       - stop animation
'info'       - display help info
'close'      - close graphics window

P.G. Bonanni / Irfan Ali  7/17/00
```

---

```
DRAWMAP - Draw a map using a rectangular grid
projection.
handle = drawmap(map[,range,s])

Draws that portion of 'map' which lies within the
geographical area specified by 'range', where 'map' is
an [N,2] matrix of contiguous (elon,nlat) pairs
separated by "pen-up" indicators (i.e., the pair "NaN
NaN"). Units for (elon,nlat) are east longitude degrees
and north latitude degrees, respectively. Parameter
'range' is a 1x4 vector whose format is like the MATLAB
'axis' parameter with x range referring to east
longitude degrees and y range to north latitude degrees.
Parameter 's' specifies the line type for the plot. The
output of the function is a handle to the resulting
plot.

Other usage modes:
1) drawmap(map)
   displays the full map using a solid line type.
2) drawmap(map,range)
   displays the specified range using a solid line type.
3) drawmap(map,s)
   displays the full map using the specified line type.

P.G. Bonanni
2/7/95
```

---

```
ECI2ECF2 - Pos/vel ECI to ECF transformation.
[xECF,vECF] = eci2ecf2(JT,xECI,vECI)
xECF = eci2ecf2(JT,xECI)

Converts positions x and velocities v from ECI to ECF,
given Julian time JT in days.

Parameters:
JT   - Nx1 vector of Julian times
xECI - Nx3 ECI position trajectory
vECI - Nx3 ECI velocity trajectory

ECF outputs 'xECF' and 'vECF' are Nx3.  Input parameter
'vECI' may be omitted if only a position transformation
is desired.

P.G. Bonanni
9/28/94
```

---

```
GREATARC - Great arc connecting two surface points.
[elon,nlat] = greatarc(elon1,nlat1,elon2,nlat2,npoints)

Generates longitude (deg E) and latitude (deg N)
coordinates representing the great arc connecting points
(elon1,nlat1) and (elon2,nlat2).  Parameter 'npoints'
specifies the number of points on the arc.

P.G. Bonanni
8/26/94
```

---

```
GRNWICH - Greenwich right ascension.
az = grnwich(JT)

Computes the right ascension of Greenwich (rad) given
Julian Time vector 'JT' (days).  (Algorithm from Meeus,
J., Astronomical Algorithms, p. 83-85.)

P.G. Bonanni (adapted from code by Craig Bennett)
10/31/94
```

---

```
INTREG - Intersection of two geographic regions.
[elon,nlat] = intreg(elon1,nlat1,elon2,nlat2)

Given two geographic regions bordered by the closed
sequences (elon1,nlat1) and (elon2,nlat2) where 'elon1'
```

```
and 'elon2' are vectors of east longitude degrees, and
'nlat1' and 'nlat2' are vectors of north latitude
degrees, calculate the region defined by the
intersection.  Assumes close sampling of the border
contours, and that both the input regions and the
intersection region have the property that great circle
arcs directed outward from their geographic centers
intersect their boundaries only once.

P.G. Bonanni (adapted from code by Irfan Ali)
7/10/00
```

---

```
KEPL2ECI - Keplerian to ECI transformation.
[xECI,vECI] = kepl2eci(a,e,i,o,w,v)

Calculates the Nx3 position trajectory 'xECI' and Nx3
velocity trajectory 'vECI' in Earth-centered-inertial
coordinates given Keplerian orbit element Nx1 sequences
(a,e,i,o,w,v).  Scalar values for any of the inputs are
acceptable.  Units for 'xECI' and 'vECI' are km and
km/sec, respectively.

The Keplerian elements are:
a  :  semimajor axis (km)
e  :  eccentricity (unitless)
i  :  inclination (rad)
o  :  right ascension of the
       ascending node (rad)
w  :  argument of perigee (rad)
v  :  true anomaly (rad)

P.G. Bonanni
3/10/95
```

---

```
LONLAT - Calculate longitude, latitude, and range.
[elon,nlat,range] = lonlat(x)

Given an Nx3 vector 'x' of Earth-fixed Cartesian
positions, calculate Nx1 input vectors specifying
longitude, latitude, and range.  Longitude 'elon' is
specified in east degrees and latitude in north degrees.
Ouput 'range' has units to match those of input
trajectory 'x'.

P.G. Bonanni
6/28/00
```

---

```
ORBITPER - Calculate period for terrestrial orbits.
T = orbitper(a)

Calculates orbital period as a function of semi-major
axis for a body in Earth orbit.  The semi-major axis 'a'
is specified in km (vector input is permitted).  Orbit
period is returned in units of seconds.

P.G. Bonanni
3/7/95
```

---

```
PERIMVIS - Calculate perimeter of visible ground region.
[elon,nlat] = perimvis(x [, elev], npoints)

Calculates a length 'npoints' sequence of (elon,nlat)
pairs that define the perimeter of the region on the
Earth's surface visible from a given position 'x' in
space.  Visibility is defined by the criterion that the
elevation to the point 'x' from the ground is greater
than or equal to angle 'elev'.  This angle is given in
degrees, and defaults to zero if omitted from the
argument list.  The position 'x' is specified in km with
respect to Earth-centered coordinates.  Units for 'elon'
and 'nlat' are east longitude degrees and north latitude
degrees, respectively.

P.G. Bonanni
6/22/00
```

---

```
POSLLR - Calculate position given longitude, latitude,
and range.
x = posllr(elon,nlat [,range])

Calculates an Nx3 vector 'x' of Earth-fixed Cartesian
positions given Nx1 input vectors specifying longitude,
latitude, and range.  Longitude 'elon' is specified in
east degrees and latitude in north degrees.  If 'range'
parameter is omitted, Earth radius is assumed.

P.G. Bonanni
3/7/95
```

---

```
PVDEG - Principal value in degrees.
```

angle1 = pvdeg(angle)

This function converts angles outside the range [0,360] to their equivalent in that range. Both scalar and matrix inputs are valid.

P.G. Bonanni
10/31/94

---

PVDEGS - Symmetric principal value in degrees.
angle1 = pvdegs(angle)

This function converts angles outside the range [-180,180] to their equivalent in that range. Both scalar and matrix inputs are valid.

P.G. Bonanni
10/31/94

---

PVRAD - Principal value in radians.
angle1 = pvrad(angle)

This function converts angles outside the range [0,2*pi] to their equivalent in that range. Both scalar and matrix inputs are valid.

P.G. Bonanni
11/10/94

---

PVRADS - Symmetric principal value in radians.
angle1 = pvrads(angle)

This function converts angles outside the range [-pi,pi] to their equivalent in that range. Both scalar and matrix inputs are valid.

P.G. Bonanni
11/10/94

---

ROT3X - 3-space rotation matrix - x.
R = rot3x(theta)

Computes the 3x3 matrix representing a rotation about the x-axis by angle 'theta'.

P.G. Bonanni
11/10/94

---

ROT3Y - 3-space rotation matrix - y.
R = rot3y(theta)

Computes the 3x3 matrix representing a rotation about the y-axis by angle 'theta'.

P.G. Bonanni
11/10/94

---

ROT3Z - 3-space rotation matrix - z.
R = rot3z(theta)

Computes the 3x3 matrix representing a rotation about the z-axis by angle 'theta'.

P.G. Bonanni
11/10/94

---

ROTATE3X - Rotate a 3-space trajectory about the x-axis.
[x1,y1,z1] = rotate3x(x,y,z,theta)

Rotates the 3-space trajectory [x,y,z] by an amount 'theta' radians about the x-axis, where 'theta' is a vector equal in size to 'x', 'y', and 'z'. Scalar inputs are extended to vectors if needed.

P.G. Bonanni
3/5/96

---

ROTATE3Y - Rotate a 3-space trajectory about the y-axis.
[x1,y1,z1] = rotate3y(x,y,z,theta)

Rotates the 3-space trajectory [x,y,z] by an amount 'theta' radians about the y-axis, where 'theta' is a vector equal in size to 'x', 'y', and 'z'. Scalar inputs are extended to vectors if needed.

P.G. Bonanni
3/5/96

---

```
ROTATE3Z - Rotate a 3-space trajectory about the z-axis.
[x1,y1,z1] = rotate3z(x,y,z,theta)

Rotates the 3-space trajectory [x,y,z] by an amount
'theta' radians about the z-axis, where 'theta' is a
vector equal in size to 'x', 'y', and 'z'.  Scalar
inputs are extended to vectors if needed.

P.G. Bonanni
3/5/96
```

---

```
STR2JT - Convert date-time string to Julian Time.
jt = str2jt(line)

Converts a date-time string to Julian time, in days.
Julian days are a continuous count of days starting from
noon Universal Time on January 1 of the year 4713 BC, a
reference useful in astronomical formulas.  Input 'line'
is a string variable having any of the following
formats:

    FORMAT                    EXAMPLE
    ------                    -------
   'dd-mmm-yyyy HH:MM:SS'     01-Mar-1995 15:45:17
   'dd-mmm-yyyy'              01-Mar-1995
   'mm/dd/yy'                 03/01/95
   'mm/dd'                    03/01
   'mmmyy'                    Mar95
   'HH:MM:SS'                 15:45:17
   'HH:MM:SS PM'               3:45:17 PM
   'HH:MM'                    15:45
   'HH:MM PM'                  3:45 PM

(Variations on date and time can be combined.)

P.G. Bonanni
7/19/00
```

---

```
SWATH - Calculate swath of visibility for an orbit.
[elon,nlat] = swath(xECF,vECF [,elev])

Generates a sequence of (elon,nlat) pairs that define
the swath of coverage for a satellite with the given
orbit.  Coverage is defined by the criterion that the
elevation to the satellite from the ground is greater
```

than or equal to angle 'elev' in degrees. Units for 'elon' and 'nlat' are east longitude degrees and north latitude degrees, respectively. The NX3 orbital position trajectory 'xECF' and velocity trajectory 'vECF' are specified in km and km/sec respectively, with respect to Earth-centered-fixed coordinates. Elevation 'elev' may be scalar or Nx1 corresponding to the orbit length. If omitted entirely, zero is assumed.

P.G. Bonanni (adapted from code by Irfan Ali)
6/29/00

---

UCOMPASS - Calculate compass directions.
[east,north,zenith] = ucompass(elon0,nlat0)

Calculates 3x1 unit vectors 'east', 'north', and 'zenith' representing the corresponding local directions for a given longitude 'elon0' and latitude 'nlat' expressed in the ECF frame. Input units are degrees east and degrees north, respectively.

P.G. Bonanni
3/8/95

---

WALKER - Generate a Walker satellite constellation.
[XECI,VECI] = walker(nsat,radius,inclin,nplanes,...
                     harmonic,ran0,anom0,time)

Generates orbit trajectories XECI = {xECI1,xECI2,...,xECInsat} and corresponding velocity trajectories VECI = {vECI1,vECI2,...,vECInsat} for a Walker satellite constellation orbiting the Earth at 'radius' km. The Walker constellation is specified by the number of satellites 'nsat', inclination angle 'inclin' (in degrees), number of planes 'nplanes', and harmonic factor 'harmonic'. Parameter 'ran0' specifies the right ascension of the ascending node (in degrees), and 'anom0' the initial true anomaly (in degrees), for the first satellite in the constellation. Vector 'time' (in seconds) defines the temporal spacing and duration of the trajectory points. (The initial value time(1) is referenced to 'anom0'.)

P.G. Bonanni (adapted from code by Irfan Ali)
6/28/00

# Index

**F**



**G**



**H**



**I**



**J**



**K**



**L**



**M**



**N**



**O**



**P**

CD-ROM DISCLAIMER

GPSR Compliance
The European Union's (EU) General Product Safety Regulation (GPSR) is a set of rules that requires consumer products to be safe and our obligations to ensure this.

If you have any concerns about our products, you can contact us on

ProductSafety@springernature.com

In case Publisher is established outside the EU, the EU authorized representative is:

Springer Nature Customer Service Center GmbH
Europaplatz 3
69115 Heidelberg, Germany

www.ingramcontent.com/pod-product-compliance
Ingram Content Group UK Ltd.
Pitfield, Milton Keynes, MK11 3LW, UK
UKHW012234240726
13966UKWH00003B/1087

* 9 7 8 1 4 7 5 7 8 3 8 9 6 *